Microincisional Cataract Surgery
The Art and Science

Microincisional Cataract Surgery
The Art and Science

Amar Agarwal, MS, FRCS, FRCOphth
Dr. Agarwal's Group of Eye Hospitals
and Eye Research Centre
Chennai, India

Richard L. Lindstrom, MD
Minnesota Eye Consultants
Minneapolis, MN

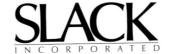

www.slackbooks.com

ISBN: 978-1-55642-943-9

Copyright © 2010 by SLACK Incorporated

All rights reserved. No part of this book may be reproduced, stored in a retrieval system or transmitted in any form or by any means, electronic, mechanical, photocopying, recording or otherwise, without written permission from the publisher, except for brief quotations embodied in critical articles and reviews.

The procedures and practices described in this book should be implemented in a manner consistent with the professional standards set for the circumstances that apply in each specific situation. Every effort has been made to confirm the accuracy of the information presented and to correctly relate generally accepted practices. The authors, editor, and publisher cannot accept responsibility for errors or exclusions or for the outcome of the material presented herein. There is no expressed or implied warranty of this book or information imparted by it. Care has been taken to ensure that drug selection and dosages are in accordance with currently accepted/recommended practice. Due to continuing research, changes in government policy and regulations, and various effects of drug reactions and interactions, it is recommended that the reader carefully review all materials and literature provided for each drug, especially those that are new or not frequently used. Any review or mention of specific companies or products is not intended as an endorsement by the author or publisher.

SLACK Incorporated uses a review process to evaluate submitted material. Prior to publication, educators or clinicians provide important feedback on the content that we publish. We welcome feedback on this work.

Published by: SLACK Incorporated
6900 Grove Road
Thorofare, NJ 08086 USA
Telephone: 856-848-1000
Fax: 856-853-5991
www.slackbooks.com

Contact SLACK Incorporated for more information about other books in this field or about the availability of our books from distributors outside the United States.

Library of Congress Cataloging-in-Publication Data

Microincisional cataract surgery : the art and science / [edited by] Amar Agarwal, Richard L. Lindstrom.
 p. ; cm.
 Includes bibliographical references and index.
 ISBN 978-1-55642-943-9 (alk. paper)
 1. Cataract–Surgery. 2. Phacoemulsification. I. Agarwal, Amar. II. Lindstrom, Richard L.
 [DNLM: 1. Phacoemulsification–methods. 2. Intraoperative Complications–therapy. 3. Lens Implantation, Intraocular–methods. 4. Microsurgery–methods.]
 RE451.M46 2010
 617.7'42059–dc22
 2009053866

For permission to reprint material in another publication, contact SLACK Incorporated. Authorization to photocopy items for internal, personal, or academic use is granted by SLACK Incorporated provided that the appropriate fee is paid directly to Copyright Clearance Center. Prior to photocopying items, please contact the Copyright Clearance Center at 222 Rosewood Drive, Danvers, MA 01923 USA; phone: 978-750-8400; website: www.copyright.com; email: info@copyright.com

Printed in the United States of America.

Last digit is print number: 10 9 8 7 6 5 4 3 2 1

DEDICATION

This book is dedicated to
a great friend,
GRAHAM BARRETT.
—*Amar Agarwal*

This book is dedicated to my wife,
JACI M. LINDSTROM.
—*Richard L. Lindstrom*

CONTENTS

Dedication .... *v*
Acknowledgments .... *ix*
About the Editors .... *xi*
Contributing Authors .... *xiii*
Preface .... *xvii*
Foreword by David F. Chang, MD .... *xix*
Introduction .... *xxi*

SECTION I: INTRODUCTION

Chapter 1: Phacoemulsification: The Machine and Technique 3
William J. Fishkind, MD, FACS

Chapter 2: Wound Architecture, Induced Astigmatism, and Aberrations in MICS and In Vivo Analysis of 700-µm Cataract Surgery 13
Dhivya Ashok Kumar, MD; Gaurav Prakash, MS; Vidya Nair, MD; and Amar Agarwal, MS, FRCS, FRCOphth

Chapter 3: Air Pump, Gas-Forced Infusion, and Fluidics 23
Smita Narsimhan, FERC; Prashaant Chaudhry, MD; Hiroshi Tsuneoka, MD; and Amar Agarwal, MS, FRCS, FRCOphth

SECTION II: MACHINES AND INSTRUMENTATION

Chapter 4: Instruments for MICS 37
L. Felipe Vejarano, MD

Chapter 5: MICS Using Torsional Phacoemulsification and the Alcon INFINITI Vision System 45
Khiun F. Tjia, MD

Chapter 6: 1.8-mm Coaxial MICS With the Stellaris Platform 61
Terence M. Devine, MD

Chapter 7: MICS and the Abbott Medical Optics Platform 71
George H. H. Beiko, BM, BCh (Oxon), FRCSC

SECTION III: MICS—SURGICAL TECHNIQUES

Chapter 8: Transition to Microincisional Cataract Surgery 89
Uday Devgan, MD, FACS, FRCS(Glasg)

Chapter 9: Microcoaxial Phacoemulsification 95
Vaishali Vasavada, MS; Viraj A. Vasavada, MS; Abhay R. Vasavada, MS, FRCS; and Shetal M. Raj, DO, MS

Chapter 10: Sub-2-mm Lens Surgery 105
Richard Packard, MD, DO, FRCS, FRCOphth

CONTENTS

Chapter 11: Three-Port Bimanual Sleeveless Microphacoemulsification Using the "Tilt and Tumble" Technique...113
Dennis C. Lu, MD; Elizabeth A. Davis, MD; David R. Hardten, MD; and Richard L. Lindstrom, MD

Chapter 12: No-Anesthesia Sub-1-mm (700-μm) Microincisional Cataract Surgery—Microphakonit 125
Athiya Agarwal, MD, DO; Soosan Jacob, MS, FRCS, FERC, Dip NB; and Amar Agarwal, MS, FRCS, FRCOphth

Chapter 13: Use of Bimanual MICS for Difficult and Challenging Cases 133
I. Howard Fine, MD; Richard S. Hoffman, MD; and Mark Packer, MD, FACS

Chapter 14: Microincisional Cataract Surgery for Pediatric Cataracts 143
Arturo Pèrez-Arteaga, MD

Chapter 15: Microincisional Cataract Surgery Combined With Other Surgeries 149
Archana Nair, MS; Dhivya Ashok Kumar, MD; and Amar Agarwal, MS, FRCS, FRCOphth

SECTION IV: MICROINCISIONAL LENSES AND COMPLICATION MANAGEMENT

Chapter 16: MICS Injector Systems 157
Kelly J. Grimes, MS and Bonnie An Henderson, MD

Chapter 17: Microincisional Intraocular Lenses 165
Mayank A. Nanavaty, DO, MRCOphth, MRCS(Ed) and David J. Spalton, FRCP, FRCS, FRCOphth

Chapter 18: Microincisional Cataract Surgery in the Era of Refractive Cataract Surgery..173
Robert Weinstock, MD and Neel R. Desai, MD

Chapter 19: Posterior Capsular Rupture and Its Management................................... 183
Soosan Jacob, MS, FRCS, FERC, Dip NB; Dhivya Ashok Kumar, MD; Kaladevi Satish, MS; Clement K. Chan, MD, FACS; and Amar Agarwal, MS, FRCS, FRCOphth

Financial Disclosures... 195
Index.. 197

ACKNOWLEDGMENTS

Nothing in this world moves without Him, and so also this book was only written by Him.

ABOUT THE EDITORS

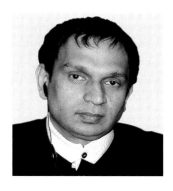

Amar Agarwal, MS, FRCS, FRCOphth is the pioneer of phakonit, which is Phako with a needle incision technology. This technique became popularized as bimanual phaco, microincision cataract surgery (MICS), or microphaco. He was the first to remove cataracts through a 0.7-mm tip with a technique called *microphakonit*. He has also discovered no anesthesia cataract surgery and FAVIT, a new technique used to remove dropped nuclei. The air pump, which was a simple idea of using an aquarium fish pump to increase the fluid into the eye in bimanual phaco and co-axial phaco, has helped prevent surge. This built the basis of various techniques of forced infusion for small incision cataract surgery. He was also the first to use trypan blue for staining epiretinal membranes and publishing the details in his 4-volume textbook of ophthalmology. He has also discovered a new refractive error called *aberropia*. He was the first to do a combined surgery of microphakonit (700 micron cataract surgery) with a 25-gauge vitrectomy in the same patient, thus having the smallest incisions possible for cataract and vitrectomy. He is also the first surgeon to implant a new mirror telescopic IOL (LMI) for patients suffering from age-related macular degeneration. He was also the first in the world to implant a glued IOL. In this technique, a PC IOL is fixed in an eye without any capsules using fibrin glue. The Malyugin ring for small pupil cataract surgery was also modified by him as the Agarwal modification of the Malyugin ring for miotic pupil cataract surgeries with posterior capsular defects. Dr. Agarwal's Eye Hospital has also done (for the first time) an Anterior segment transplantation in a 4-month-old child with anterior staphyloma.

Professor Agarwal has received many awards for his work done in ophthalmology, the most significant being the Barraquer Award and the Kelman Award. His videos have won many awards at the film festivals of ASCRS, AAO, and ESCRS. He has also written more than 50 books, which have been published in English, Spanish, and Polish. He also trains doctors from all over the world on phaco, bimanual phaco, LASIK, and retina. He heads Dr. Agarwal's Group of Eye Hospitals, which has 30 eye hospitals. He is also Professor of Ophthalmology at Ramachandra Medical College in Chennai, India.

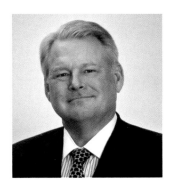

Richard L. Lindstrom, MD is founder and attending surgeon at Minnesota Eye Consultants and Adjunct Professor Emeritus at the University of Minnesota Department of Ophthalmology. He is a board-certified ophthalmologist and internationally recognized leader in corneal, cataract, refractive, and laser surgery. He has been at the forefront of ophthalmology's evolutionary changes throughout his career as a recognized researcher, teacher, inventor, writer, lecturer, and highly acclaimed physician and surgeon.

After graduating Magna Cum Laude from the College of Liberal Arts at the University of Minnesota, Dr. Lindstrom completed his doctorate degree in medicine in 1972. He conducted research, residency, and fellowship training in cornea at the University of Minnesota and affiliated hospitals. He extended his anterior segment surgery fellowship training at Mary Shiels Hospital in Dallas, TX and was a Heed fellow in glaucoma at

ABOUT THE EDITORS

University Hospital in Salt Lake City, UT. In 1980, Dr. Lindstrom returned to the University of Minnesota, where he spent 10 years on the faculty of the Department of Ophthalmology, the last 2 as a full professor and the Harold G. Scheie Research Chair. He continues as Adjunct Professor Emeritus, Chairman of the Vision Foundation, and Associate Director of the Minnesota Lions Eye Bank at the University of Minnesota. He entered private practice in 1989 and has led the growth and expansion of Minnesota Eye Consultants, serving as managing partner for 15 years.

Dr. Lindstrom is medical director of Sightpath Medical, which includes MSS and Laser Vision. He is also medical director of Refractec. He is Chief Medical Editor of the USA and International editions of *Ocular Surgery News*, which reaches 82,000 ophthalmologists worldwide.

Dr. Lindstrom is past President of the American Society of Cataract and Refractive Surgeons. He serves on the Executive Committee and is the Chair of the ASCRS Foundation. He is also past President of the International Society of Refractive Surgery, the International Intraocular Implant Club, and the International Refractive Surgery Club. He is the Global Education Liaison of the International Society of Refractive Surgery of the American Academy of Ophthalmology. He is Chairman and CEO of Lindstrom Restoration, a 3-generation family business. He has endowed funds supporting the University of Minnesota Department of Ophthalmology, the Eye Bank Association of America, and the University of Minnesota Tennis Team.

Dr. Lindstrom holds over 35 patents in ophthalmology and has developed a number of solutions, intraocular lenses, and instruments that are used in clinical practices globally. He serves on the Board of Directors of AcuFocus, Inc, TLC Vision, Occulogix, Refractec, the Minnesota Medical Foundation, and Inner City Tennis.

A frequent lecturer throughout the world on cornea, cataract, and refractive surgery, he has presented over 40 named lectures and keynote speeches before professional societies in the US and abroad, giving the Blumenthal Memorial Lecture in Jerusalem, Israel; the Benedetto Strampelli Medal Lecture in Rome, Italy; the Albrecht von Garefe-Vorlesung Innovator's Lecture in Nuremberg, Germany; IIIC Medal Lecture in Berlin, Germany; and the Susrata Lecture in Baltimore, MD.

Dr. Lindstrom serves on a number of journal editorial boards, including *JCRS*, *JRS*, and *Ophthalmic Surgery*. He is the Honorary Editor-in-Chief of the US/Chinese *Journal of Ophthalmology*. He has co-edited 7 books and published over 350 peer-reviewed journal articles and 60 book chapters. His professional affiliations are extensive, including Liaison of the International Society of Refractive Surgery of the American Academy of Ophthalmology.

He is the recipient of numerous awards for distinguished service by national and international ophthalmology associations, including the LANS, Barraquer, and the first lifetime achievement award from the International Society of Refractive Surgery in October 1995. He also was honored with another lifetime achievement award in October 2002; the Binkhorst Lecture Award from the American Society of Cataract and Refractive Surgery; the Bausch & Lomb Lifetime Achievement Award in April 2005; the Benjamin F. Boyd Humanitarian Award in August 2000; and the Paton Award and NACT from the Eye Bank Association of America.

CONTRIBUTING AUTHORS

Athiya Agarwal, MD, DO (Chapter 12)
Consultant
Dr. Agarwal's Group of Eye Hospitals and Eye Research Centre
Chennai, India

George H. H. Beiko, BM, BCh (Oxon), FRCSC (Chapter 7)
Assistant Professor, Surgery (Ophthalmology)
McMaster University
Lecturer, Ophthalmology
University of Toronto
Saint Catharines, Canada

Clement K. Chan, MD, FACS (Chapter 19)
Medical Director, Southern California Desert Retina Consultants, M.C.
Inland Retina Consultants
Palm Springs, CA
Associate Clinical Professor, Ophthalmology
Loma Linda University
Loma Linda, CA

Prashaant Chaudhry, MD (Chapter 3)
Consultant
Dr. Agarwal's Group of Eye Hospitals and Eye Research Centre
Chennai, India

Elizabeth A. Davis, MD (Chapter 11)
Minnesota Eye Consultants
Minneapolis, MN

Neel R. Desai, MD (Chapter 18)
Cornea, Cataract and Refractive Specialist
Eye Institute of West Florida
St. Petersburg, FL

Uday Devgan, MD, FACS, FRCS(Glasg) (Chapter 8)
Medical Director and Chief Surgeon
Devgan Eye Center for Cataract & Refractive Surgery
Chief of Ophthalmology
Olive View UCLA Medical Center
Associate Clinical Professor, Ophthalmology
Jules Stein Eye Institute
UCLA School of Medicine
Los Angeles, CA

Terence M. Devine, MD (Chapter 6)
Chief of Ophthalmology
Guthrie Clinic
Sayre, PA
Associate Professor, Ophthalmology
State University of New York
Albany, NY

I. Howard Fine, MD (Chapter 13)
Clinical Professor, Ophthalmology
Casey Eye Institute
Oregon Health & Science University
Portland, OR
Co-founder, Oregon Eye Institute and the Oregon Eye Surgery Center
Private Practice, Drs. Fine, Hoffman & Packer, LLC
Eugene, OR

William J. Fishkind, MD, FACS (Chapter 1)
Clinical Professor, Ophthalmology
University of Utah
Salt Lake City, UT
Clinical Instructor, Ophthalmology
University of Arizona
Co-Director, Fishkind, Bakewell, & Maltzman Eye Care and Surgery Center
Tucson, AZ

Kelly J. Grimes, MS (Chapter 16)
Harvard Medical School
Clinical Research Associate
Massachusetts Eye and Ear Infirmary
Boston, MA

David R. Hardten, MD (Chapter 11)
Director of Fellowships
Minnesota Eye Consultants
Adjunct Associate Professor, Ophthalmology
University of Minnesota
Minneapolis, MN

Bonnie An Henderson, MD (Chapter 16)
Partner, Ophthalmic Consultants of Boston
Assistant Clinical Professor, Ophthalmology
Harvard Medical School
Boston, MA

CONTRIBUTING AUTHORS

Richard S. Hoffman, MD (Chapter 13)
Clinical Associate Professor, Ophthalmology
Casey Eye Institute
Oregon Health & Science University
Portland, OR
Private Practice, Drs. Fine, Hoffman & Packer, LLC
Eugene, OR

Soosan Jacob, MS, FRCS, FERC, Dip NB (Chapters 12 and 19)
Consultant
Dr. Agarwal's Group of Eye Hospitals and Eye Research Centre
Chennai, India

Dhivya Ashok Kumar, MD (Chapter 2, Chapter 15, Chapter 19)
Consultant
Dr. Agarwal's Group of Eye Hospitals and Eye Research Centre
Chennai, India

Dennis C. Lu, MD (Chapter 11)
Kaiser Permanente
West Los Angeles Medical Center
Department of Ophthalmology
Los Angeles, CA

Archana Nair, MS (Chapter 15)
Consultant
Dr. Agarwal's Group of Eye Hospitals and Eye Research Centre
Chennai, India

Vidya Nair, MD (Chapter 2)
Consultant
Dr. Agarwal's Group of Eye Hospitals and Eye Research Centre
Chennai, India

Mayank A. Nanavaty, DO, MRCOphth, MRCS(Ed) (Chapter 17)
Research Fellow
Department of Ophthalmology
St. Thomas' Hospital
London, UK

Smita Narsimhan, FERC (Chapter 3)
Consultant
Dr. Agarwal's Group of Eye Hospitals and Eye Research Centre
Chennai, India

Richard Packard, MD, DO, FRCS, FRCOphth (Chapter 10)
Senior Consultant Surgeon
Prince Charles Eye Unit
King Edward VII Hospital
Windsor, England

Mark Packer, MD, FACS (Chapter 13)
Clinical Associate Professor, Ophthalmology
Casey Eye Institute
Oregon Health & Science University
Portland, OR
Private Practice, Drs. Fine, Hoffman & Packer, LLC
Eugene, OR

Arturo Pèrez-Arteaga, MD (Chapter 14)
Assistant Professor, Medical Basic Sciences
Facultad de Estudios Profesionales
Iztacala, Mexico
Universidad Nacional Autonoma de México
Medical Director, Centro Oftalmológico Tlalnepantla
Tlalnepantla, Mexico

Gaurav Prakash, MS (Chapter 2)
Consultant
Dr. Agarwal's Group of Eye Hospitals and Eye Research Centre
Chennai, India

Shetal M. Raj, DO, MS (Chapter 9)
Iladevi Cataract & IOL Research Centre
Raghudeep Eye Clinic
Memnagar, Ahmedabad, India

Kaladevi Satish, MS (Chapter 19)
Consultant
Dr. Agarwal's Group of Eye Hospitals and Eye Research Centre
Chennai, India

CONTRIBUTING AUTHORS

David J. Spalton, FRCP, FRCS, FRCOphth (Chapter 17)
Consultant Ophthalmologist
Department of Ophthalmology
St. Thomas' Hospital
London, UK

Khiun F. Tjia, MD (Chapter 5)
Isala Clinics
Zwolle, The Netherlands

Hiroshi Tsuneoka, MD (Chapter 3)
Professor and Chairman
Department of Ophthalmology
Jikei University School of Medicine
Tokyo, Japan

Abhay R. Vasavada, MS, FRCS (Chapter 9)
Iladevi Cataract & IOL Research Centre
Raghudeep Eye Clinic
Memnagar, Ahmedabad, India

Vaishali Vasavada, MS (Chapter 9)
Iladevi Cataract & IOL Research Centre
Raghudeep Eye Clinic
Memnagar, Ahmedabad, India

Viraj A. Vasavada, MS (Chapter 9)
Iladevi Cataract & IOL Research Centre
Raghudeep Eye Clinic
Memnagar, Ahmedabad, India

L. Felipe Vejarano, MD (Chapter 4)
Department of Ophthalmology
Universidad del Cauca
Chief of Surgery
Fundación Oftalmológica Vejarano
Popayán, Colombia

Robert Weinstock, MD (Chapter 18)
Director, Cataract and Refractive Surgery
Eye Institute of West Florida
Associate Clinical Professor, Department of Ophthalmology
University of South Florida
St. Petersburg, FL

PREFACE

Since phakonit was started in 1998, so many changes have occurred in microincision cataract surgery (MICS). Now with biaxial and coaxial MICS, one can perform any type of cataract surgery. Microincision lenses have also come of age. Companies have started making special machines and instruments for MICS. Today we are able to perform 700-μm cataract surgery with this technique. Looking at all of this, we thought that a book on this new, evolving surgical technique was essential.

This book covers the evolution of MICS, MICS techniques, wound morphology, and machines and instruments used in MICS. It also includes sections explaining the surgical techniques one can perform in challenging cases with MICS. Most important of all is the final section, which deals with the management of intraoperative complications.

This book would not be possible without the help of the excellent contributors who have spent their time and energy in preparing each chapter. Certain people who helped us along the way were Dr. Dhivya Ashok Kumar and Brenda L. Boff. The entire team at SLACK, starting with John Bond, Jennifer Briggs, Michelle Gatt, Dani Karaszkiewicz, and others, stood with us and guided us along the way. We will always be grateful to each one of them.

In the end, dear reader, we hope you enjoy reading this book as much as we enjoyed writing it.

Professor Amar Agarwal
Dr. Richard L. Lindstrom

FOREWORD

The past several years have seen renewed interest in further downsizing incisions for cataract surgery. This is a logical continuation down a path that Charlie Kelman started us on more than 3 decades ago. Thanks to innovations in ultrasound power modulation, fluidics, instrumentation, and technique, microincisional phaco has evolved into a safe and efficient procedure within a relatively short period of time. We are now gaining access to advanced foldable IOL technologies that allow us to fully capitalize on the parallel improvements in microincisional phaco technique and technology.

This well-illustrated surgical textbook is the most comprehensive and authoritative review of the current "state of the art" of microincisional cataract surgery (MICS). It appropriately provides detailed coverage of the latest phaco and IOL technology, as well as the multitude of advanced techniques for both coaxial and biaxial MICS. Editors Amar Agarwal and Dick Lindstrom are both renowned surgical innovators who were among the earliest pioneers in MICS. They have assembled an exceptional faculty of experts, who also excel as educators in this dynamic field.

Once phacoemulsification took hold as the dominant cataract procedure in the 1990s, the quest to further reduce incision size focused on alternatives to ultrasound. Novel and promising approaches have included Erbium and YAG laser phaco, phacotemesis, sonics, Catarex, and AquaLase. The irony is that after all of this innovative research and experimentation, the best modality for removing a lens in 2010 is still ultrasound. It is quite remarkable that in this era of rapidly advancing medical technology, we are still using essentially the same ultrasound instrumentation—coaxial irrigating sleeve and all—that Charlie Kelman first dreamed up in the late 1960s. In all of medicine, such a situation must be truly unique.

With new technological advances arriving at such a rapid rate, it is a remarkably exciting time to be a cataract surgeon. This wonderful textbook is an appropriate way to celebrate and advance the progress and promise of microincisional cataract surgery.

David F. Chang, MD
Clinical Professor
University of California
San Francisco, CA
Altos Eye Physicians
Los Altos, CA

INTRODUCTION

MICS: From Phakonit to Microphakonit

Amar Agarwal, MS, FRCS, FRCOphth

When phakonit was started in 1998,[1] I did not realize it would become so popular so fast. I wish I could say it was a brilliant invention of mine, but I cannot. The reason is that this invention (as do all inventions and discoveries) came as a message to me from the Almighty and so the invention is His and only His.

How it all Started

I am basically a vitreoretinal surgeon and used to do all lensectomies with the phaco handpiece. I did not have a fragmatome, so I used to remove the infusion sleeve and pass the phaco needle into the lens through the pars plana. Infusion would be through the infusion cannula, which is connected in all vitrectomies. In this way, I could remove the cataracts in patients who then required vitrectomy for proliferative vitreo-retinopathy or any other posterior segment pathology.

I subsequently began to think about using this system for cataracts for the anterior segment surgeon. The problem was how to have an irrigation system present inside the eye. In 1998, the thought of taking a needle, bending it like a chopper, and using that for irrigation and chopping occurred to me. I realized that a corneal burn could occur, which led to the concept of irrigating the corneal wound from outside. In the first case on August 15, 1998, I removed the infusion sleeve from the phaco handpiece and connected a 20-gauge needle to the irrigation bottle, then bent the needle of the needle holder in such a way that it could also be used for chopping. Understandably, when I bent the needle like that it obviously did not come out very well. Another problem with using a needle was the bevel; if I pulled the needle out a little bit, the bevel was outside the eye and the chamber would collapse. For the incision, I used the Micro vitreoretinal blade (MVR blade), which vitreoretinal surgeons use for vitrectomies. This does not create the perfect valve as with the diamond and sapphire knives of today, but that was enough at that time.

When I had finished the rhexis, I knew the hydrodissection was tricky because the incision size was much smaller, and so the amount of fluid escaping from the eye would not be much. Avoiding a lot of fluid when hydrodissecting can prevent a dropped nucleus.

During surgery, I realized I was having a lot of anterior chamber shallowing. Whenever I would start to remove the nucleus, the chamber would partially collapse. It was obvious that the amount of fluid entering the eye was not enough compared to the amount exiting the eye, so I stopped the surgery and shifted to an 18-gauge needle. To my surprise, everything went well after that. Even though chopping the hard cataract was not as easy as it is now with a chopper, I knew that with more refined instruments, this surgical technique would work. I was convinced that this could be the next frontier in cataract surgery because the incision size was reduced drastically.

NO ANESTHESIA CATARACT SURGERY

On June 13, 1998, in Ahmedabad, India, I performed the first live no anesthesia cataract surgery for a workshop organized by the Indian Intraocular Implant and Refractive Society. Later on we did a study that was subsequently published in the *Journal of Cataract and Refractive Surgery*.[2,3]

> On August 22, 1998, the first live surgery of phakonit was done in Pune, India for the Indian Intraocular Implant and Refractive Society conference.

AIR PUMP

One of the main problems in phakonit was the fluidics. As explained earlier, the amount of fluid entering the eye was less than the amount of fluid exiting the eye. Dr. Sunita Agarwal understood this problem and started pushing air into the infusion bottle to get more pressurized fluid out of the bottle.[4] When it worked, she then took an aquarium air pump and connected it to the infusion bottle via an IV set. This gave a constant supply of air into the infusion bottle and the amount of fluid coming out of the irrigating chopper was quite enough for us to move from an 18-gauge irrigating chopper to a 20- or 21-gauge irrigating chopper. This was the first time pressurized fluid was used in anterior segment surgeries. In 2009, Bausch & Lomb (Aliso Viejo, CA) installed the air pump in their Stellaris machine to give good control of the pressurized infusion system.

MICROINCISIONAL CATARACT SURGERY

In 1985, Steve Shearing published a paper on separating the infusion from the phaco handpiece.[5] T. Hara from Japan also did the same in 1987.[6] I had not heard of any of this

> In 1999:
> * P. Crozafon reported the successful use of a sleeveless 21-gauge Teflon-coated tip for minimally invasive bimanual phaco.
> * Hiroshi Tseunoka from Japan[7,8] studied the use of ultrasonic phacoemulsification and aspiration for lens extraction through a microincision.
>
> In 2000:
> * Jorge Alio from Spain[9] coined the term *MICS* or microincisional cataract surgery. This meant cataract surgery could be done through a 2.0-mm incision or less. This included laser cataract surgery and ultrasound (phakonit).
> * Randall Olson was the first to resurrect interest in the United Stated and then to do studies published in peer review journals to answer the concerns of early critics.[10-13] He termed it *microphaco*.

EVOLUTION OF ANESTHETIC TECHNIQUES OF CATARACT SURGERY

Technique	Year	Author/Surgeon
General anesthesia	1846	---
Topical cocaine	1881	Koller
Injectable cocaine	1884	Knapp
Retrobulbar (4% cocaine)	1884	Knapp
Orbicularis akinesia	1914	Van Lint, O'Briens Atkinson
Hyaluridinase	1948	Atkinson
Posterior peribulbar	1985	Davis & Mandel
Limbal	1990	Furata et al
Anterior peribulbar	1991	Bloomberg
Pinpoint anesthesia	1992	Fukasawa
Topical	1992	Fichman
Topical plus intracameral	1995	Gills
No anesthesia	1998	Agarwal
Cryoanalgesia	1999	Gutierrez-Carmona
Xylocaine jelly	1999	Koch & Assia
Hypothesis, no anesthesia	2001	Pandey & Agarwal
Viscoanesthesia	2001	Werner et al

work when I started the concept of phakonit. As phakonit gradually became more popular, work done by these early pioneers were more and more appreciated.

One problem in phakonit was that there would be a spray of fluid over the cornea whenever one would do phakonit. To solve this problem, one can use the hub of the infusion sleeve—the infusion sleeve would only be over the base of the needle.[14] Using videos and a special vernier caliper, sub 1-mm phakonit surgery was documented and demonstrated using a 21-gauge irrigating chopper and a 0.8-mm phaco needle.[14]

MICS IOLs:
- Kristine Kreiner made an ultrasmall incision IOL[15] using a special co-polymer as the lens material.
- The first lens (an Acri.Smart IOL, Carl Zeiss Meditec, Jena, Germany) was implanted by Kanellopoulos in 2000.[16]
- The ThinOptX company (Abingdon, VA) headed by Wayne Callahan made an ultrathin lens using the Fresnel principles.[17,18] The first such lens was implanted by Jairo Hoyos from Spain. The second was implanted by Jorge Alio from Spain. They had heard of my work and sent me some lenses, which I then implanted after phakonit.
- I realized also that it would be better to have a smaller optic lens and designed a special 5-mm optic rollable IOL for ThinOptX, which was then made by Wayne and Scott Callahan. These were the first 5-mm optic ThinOptX rollable IOLs implanted, hence the name *rollable IOL* rather than *foldable IOL*.

EVOLUTION OF TECHNIQUES OF CATARACT SURGERY

Technique	Year	Author/Surgeon
Couching	800 BC	Susutra
ECCE* (inferior incision)	1745	J Daviel
ECCE (superior incision)	1860	Von Graefe
ICCE** (tumbling)	1880	H Smith
ECCE with PC-IOL***	1949	Sir H Ridley
ECCE with AC-IOL****	1951	B Strampelli
Phacoemulsification	1967	CD Kelman
Foldable IOLs	1984	T Marrocco
CCC	1988	HV Gimbel & T Neuhann
Hydrodissection	1992	IH Fine
In-the-bag fixation	1992	DJ Apple & IE Assia
Accommodating IOLs	1997	S Cummings & Kamman
Phakonit (Bimanual Phaco)	1998	A Agarwal
Air pump to present surgery (gas-forced infusion)	1999	S Agarwal
FAVIT technique	1999	A Agarwal
MICS terminology	2000	J Alio
Microphaco terminology and using a 0.8-mm phaco needle	2000	R Olson
Dye-enhanced cataract surgery	2000	SK Pandey et al
Sealed capsule irrigation	2001	Al Maloof
Factors for PCO prevention	2002-2004	DJ Apple et al
Microincisional co-axial phaco (MICP)	2005	Takayuki Akahoshi
Microphakonit—cataract surgery with a 0.7-mm tip	2005	A Agarwal

* ECCE = Extracapsular cataract extraction

** ICCE = Intracapsular cataract extraction

*** PC-IOL = Posterior chamber intraocular lens

**** AC-IOL = Anterior chamber intraocular lens

MICROPHAKONIT: 700 MICRON CATARACT SURGERY

In 2005, I used a 0.7-mm phaco needle tip with a 0.7-mm irrigating chopper to remove cataracts through the smallest incision possible and termed it *microphakonit* to differentiate it from *phakonit*.[19,20] When we wanted to use a 0.7-mm phaco needle, we wondered whether the needle would be able to hold the energy of the ultrasound. Larry Laks from MicroSurgical Technology (Redmond, WA) made the 0.7-mm phaco needle and 0.7-mm irrigating chopper, which I designed.

BIMANUAL PHACO/BIAXIAL PHACO

Internationally, the name for phakonit became *bimanual phaco*. The idea was to separate it from coaxial phaco in which the irrigation is with the phaco handpiece. Steve Arshinoff coined the term *biaxial phaco* to make it more understandable and separating it from co-axial phaco.[21] Biaxial accurately describes what is being done in biaxial phaco, without referencing the size of the incision (which is likely to change with time), the number of hands used for the procedure, or the size of the incision (which undoubtedly will decrease with time), irrespective of the axiality of the procedure.

MICROINCISIONAL CO-AXIAL PHACO

In 2005, Takayuki Akahoshi came out with a great concept. He designed a nano sleeve with the help of Alcon (Fort Worth, TX). The idea was to allow co-axial phaco through a sub-2-mm incision. Thus a new term was coined—*microincisional co-axial phaco* (MICP).

MICS: C-MICS AND B-MICS

The standard terminology used for all of the procedures is MICS. To differentiate MICP from bimanual phaco, the term C-MICS is used for coaxial MICS and B-MICS is used for biaxial MICS. In this book, we will use the terms coaxial or bimanual MICS.

SUMMARY

Today, phakonit or MICS has taken the ophthalmologic world by storm. The only problem right now is to get more lenses into the market that will pass through sub-1-mm incisions and at the same time not reduce the quality of vision for the patients. These must also have an excellent injector system and should be user friendly. Many surgeons and pioneers from different parts of the world have made bimanual MICS/coaxial MICS what it is today. We have come a long way in cataract surgery, but still have a long way to go.

REFERENCES

1. Agarwal A, Agarwal S, Agarwal A, Narang P, Narang S. Phakonit: phacoemulsification through a 0.9 mm incision. *J Cataract Refract Surg.* 2001;27(10):1548-1552.
2. Agarwal A, Agarwal S, Agarwal A. No anesthesia cataract surgery. In: Agarwal S, Agarwal A, Sachdev MS, Mehta KR, eds. *Phacoemulsification, Laser Cataract Surgery and Foldable IOLs.* New Delhi, India: Jaypee Brothers; 1998:144-154.
3. Pandey SK, Werner L, Apple DJ, Agarwal A, Agarwal A, Agarwal S. No-anesthesia clear corneal phacoemulsification versus topical and topical plus intracameral anesthesia: randomized clinical trial. *J Cataract Refract Surg.* 2001;27(10):1643-1650.
4. Agarwal A, Agarwal S, Agarwal A, Lal V, Patel N. Antichamber collapser. *J Cataract Refract Surg.* 2002;28(7):1085-1086.
5. Shearing S, Relyea R, Loaiza A, Shearing R. Routine phacoemulsification through a 1.0 mm non-sutured incision. *Cataract.* 1985;1:6-8.
6. Hara T, Hara T. Clinical results of phacoemulsification and complete in the bag fixation. *J Cataract and Refractive Surgery.* 1987;13;279-286.
7. Tsuenoka H, Shiba T, Takahashi Y. Feasibility of ultrasound cataract surgery with a 1.4 mm incision. *J Cataract Refract Surg.* 2001;27(6):934-940.
8. Tsuenoka H, Shiba T, Takahashi Y. Feasibility of ultrasound cataract surgery with a 1.4 mm incision: clinical results. *J Cataract Refract Surg.* 2002;28:81-86.
9. Alio J. What does MICS require in Alios textbook MICS? *Highlights of Ophthalmology.* 2004;1-4.
10. Soscia W, Howard JG, Olson RJ. Microphacoemulsification with Whitestar: a wound-temperature study. *J Cataract Refract Surg.* 2002;28(6):1044-1046.
11. Soscia W, Howard JG, Olson RJ. Bimanual phacoemulsification through 2 stab incisions: a wound-temperature study. *J Cataract Refract Surg.* 2002;28(6):1039-1043.
12. Olson RJ. Microphaco chop: rationale and technique. In: Chang DF, ed. *Phaco Chop: Mastering Techniques, Optimizing Technology, and Avoiding Complications.* Thorofare, NJ: SLACK Incorporated; 2004:227-237.
13. Chang DF. Bimanual phaco chop: fluidic strategies. In: Chang DF, ed. *Phaco Chop: Mastering Techniques, Optimizing Technology, and Avoiding Complications.* Thorofare, NJ: Slack Incorporated; 2004:239-250.
14. Agarwal A, Agarwal S, Agarwal A. Phakonit: a new technique of removing cataracts through a 0.9 mm incision. In: Agarwal S, Agarwal A, Sachdev MS, Mehta KR, eds. *Phacoemulsification, Laser Cataract Surgery and Foldable IOLs.* New Delhi, India: Jaypee Brothers; 1998:139-143.

INTRODUCTION

15. Agarwal A, Agarwal S, Agarwal A. Phakonit with an acritec IOL. *J Cataract Refract Surg*. 2003;29(4):854-855.
16. Kanellopoulos AJ. New laser system points way to ultrasmall incision cataract surgery. *Eurotimes*. 2000;5.
17. Agarwal A, Agarwal S, Agarwal A. The Phakonit ThinOptX rollable intraocular lens. In: Agarwal A, ed. *Presbyopia: A Surgical Textbook*. Thorofare, NJ: SLACK Incorporated; 2002;187-194.
18. Pandey SK, Werner L, Agarwal A, et al. Phakonit: cataract removal through a sub 1.0 mm incision with implantation of the ThinOptX rollable intraocular lens. *J Cataract Refract Surg*. 2002;28(9):1710-1713.
19. Agarwal A, Trivedi RH, Jacob S, Agarwal A, Agarwal S. Microphakonit: 700 micron cataract surgery. *Clin Ophthalmol*. 2007;1(3):323-325.
20. Agarwal A, Ashokkumar D, Jacob S, Agarwal A. In vivo analysis of wound architecture in 700 micron microphakonit surgery. *J Cataract Refract Surg*. 2008;34(9):1554-1560.
21. Arshinoff SA. Biaxial phacoemulsification. Letter. *J Cataract Refract Surg*. 2005;31(4):646.

SECTION I
INTRODUCTION

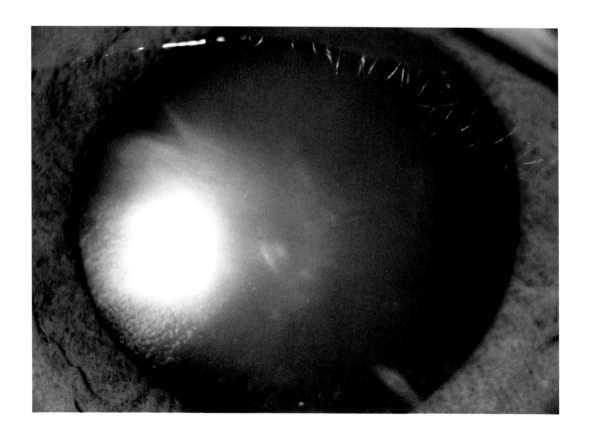

Chapter 1

Phacoemulsification: The Machine and Technique

William J. Fishkind, MD, FACS

All phaco machines consist of a computer to generate ultrasonic impulses, a transducer, and piezoelectric crystals to turn these electronic signals into mechanical energy. The energy thus created is then harnessed, within the eye, to overcome the inertia of the lens and emulsify it. Once turned into emulsate, the fluidic systems remove the emulsate, replacing it with balanced salt solution. The recent trend in phaco surgery is to minimize power utilizing new power modalities and to maximize the use of fluidics to remove the cataractous lens.[1-5]

Power Generation

Power is created by the interaction of frequency and stroke length. *Frequency* is defined as the speed of the needle movement. It is determined by the manufacturer of the machine. Presently, most machines operate at a frequency of between 35,000 cycles per second (Hz) to 45,000 cycles per second. This frequency range is the most efficient for nuclear emulsification. Lower frequencies are less efficient and higher frequencies create excess heat.

Frequency is maintained constant by tuning circuitry designed into the machine computer. Tuning is vital because the phaco tip is required to operate in varied media. For example, the resistance of the aqueous is less than the resistance of the cortex, which, in turn, is less than the resistance of the nucleus. As the resistance to the phaco tip varies, small alterations in frequency are created by the tuning circuitry in the computer to maintain maximum efficiency. The surgeon will subjectively appreciate good tuning circuitry by a sense of smoothness and power.

Stroke length is defined as the length of the needle movement. This length is generally 2 to 6 mil (thousandths of an inch). Most machines operate in the 2- to 4-mil range. Longer stroke lengths are prone to generate excess heat. The longer the stroke length, the greater the physical impact on the nucleus and the greater the generation of cavitation forces. Stroke length is determined by foot pedal excursion in position 3 during linear control of phaco.

Energy at the Phaco Tip

The actual tangible forces, which emulsify the nucleus, are thought to be a blend of the "jackhammer" effect and cavitation. The jackhammer effect is merely the physical striking of the needle against the nucleus. The cavitation effect is more convoluted. Recent studies indicate that there are 2 kinds of cavitational energy: transient cavitation and sustained cavitation.

TRANSIENT CAVITATION

The phaco needle, moving through the liquid medium of the aqueous at ultrasonic speeds, creates intense zones of high and low pressure. Low pressure, created with backward movement of the tip, literally pulls dissolved gases out of solution, thus giving rise to microbubbles. Forward tip movement then creates an equally intense zone of high pressure. This produces compression of the microbubbles until they implode. At the moment of implosion, the bubbles create a temperature of 13,000 degrees and a shock wave of 75,000 psi. Of the microbubbles created, 75% implode, amassing to create a powerful shock wave, radiating from the phaco tip in the direction of the bevel with annular spread; however, 25% of the bubbles are too large to implode. These microbubbles are swept up in the shock wave and radiate with it. Transient cavitation is a violent event. The energy created by transient cavitation exists for no more than 6 to 25 ms. It is this form of cavitation that is thought to generate the energy responsible for emulsification of cataractous material (Figure 1-1).

The cavitation energy thus created can be directed in any desired direction because the angle of the bevel of the phaco needle governs the direction of the generation of the shock wave and microbubbles.

The author has developed a method of visualization of these forces, called *enhanced cavitation*. Using this process, it can be seen that with a 45-degree tip, the cavitation wave is generated at 45 degrees from the tip and comes to a focus 1 mm from it. Similarly, a 30-degree tip generates cavitation at a 30-degree angle from the bevel, and a 15-degree tip at 15 degrees from the bevel (Figure 1-2). A 0-degree tip creates the cavitation wave directly in front of the tip and the focal point is 0.5 mm from the tip (Figure 1-3). The Kelman tip (Alcon, Fort Worth, TX) has a broad band of powerful cavitation, which radiates from the area of the angle in the shaft. A weak area of cavitation is developed from the bevel but is inconsequential.

Taking into consideration analysis of enhanced cavitation, it can be concluded that phacoemulsification is most efficient when both the jackhammer effect and cavitation energy are combined. To accomplish this, the bevel of the needle should be turned toward the nucleus or nuclear fragment. This simple maneuver will cause the broad bevel of the needle to strike the nucleus. This will enhance the physical force of the needle striking the nucleus. In addition, the cavitation force is then concentrated into the nucleus rather than away from it. Finally, in this configuration, the vacuum force can be maximally exploited as occlusion is encouraged (Figure 1-4). This causes the energy to emulsify the nucleus and be absorbed by it. A 0-degree tip automatically focuses both the jackhammer and cavitational energy directly in front of it (Figure 1-5). When the bevel is turned away from the nucleus, the cavitational energy is directed up and away from the nucleus toward the iris and endothelium (Figure 1-6).

SUSTAINED CAVITATION

If phaco energy is continued beyond 25 ms, transient cavitation with generation of microbubbles and shock waves ends. The bubbles then begin to vibrate without implosion. No shock wave is generated. Therefore, there is no emulsification energy produced. Sustained cavitation is ineffective for emulsification of the cataractous lens.

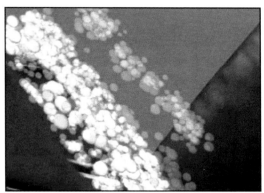

Figure 1-1. Microbubbles generated at the phaco tip. (Reprinted with permission from Agarwal A. *Phaco Nightmares: Conquering Cataract Catastrophes*. Thorofare, NJ: SLACK Incorporated; 2006.)

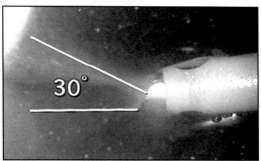

Figure 1-2. 30-degree tip. Enhanced cavitation shows ultrasonic wave focused 1 mm from the tip, spreading at an angle of 30 degrees. (Reprinted with permission from Agarwal A. *Phaco Nightmares: Conquering Cataract Catastrophes*. Thorofare, NJ: SLACK Incorporated; 2006.)

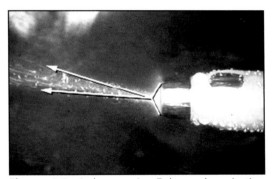

Figure 1-3. 0-degree tip. Enhanced cavitation shows ultrasonic wave focused one-half mm in front of the tip, spreading directly in front of it. (Reprinted with permission from Agarwal A. *Phaco Nightmares: Conquering Cataract Catastrophes*. Thorofare, NJ: SLACK Incorporated; 2006.)

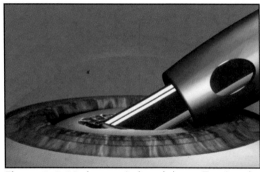

Figure 1-4. 30-degree tip bevel down. Turning the bevel of the phaco tip toward the nucleus focuses cavitation and jackhammer energy into the nucleus. (Reprinted with permission from Agarwal A. *Phaco Nightmares: Conquering Cataract Catastrophes*. Thorofare, NJ: SLACK Incorporated; 2006.)

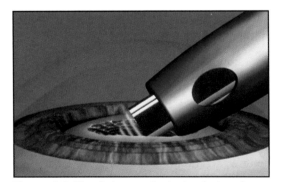

Figure 1-5. The 0-degree tip, by its design, focuses both jackhammer and cavitation forces directly ahead and into the nucleus. (Reprinted with permission from Agarwal A. *Phaco Nightmares: Conquering Cataract Catastrophes*. Thorofare, NJ: SLACK Incorporated; 2006.)

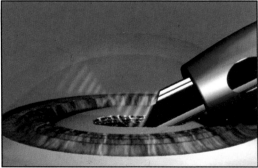

Figure 1-6. 30-degree tip, bevel up. The bevel is turned away from the nucleus. Cavitation energy is wasted and may damage the iris and endothelium. (Reprinted with permission from Agarwal A. *Phaco Nightmares: Conquering Cataract Catastrophes*. Thorofare, NJ: SLACK Incorporated; 2006.)

Water bath hydroponic studies indicate that transient cavitation is significantly more powerful than sustained cavitation. With this information in mind, it would appear that continuous phaco is best used to emulsify the intact nucleus, held in place by the capsular bag, as one does during the sculpting phase of divide-and-conquer or stop-and-chop. Transient cavitation is maximized during micropulse phaco. This is best used during phaco of the nuclear fragments in the later phase of the above 2 procedures or during phaco chop procedures.

The Alcon Aspiration Bypass System (ABS) tip modification is available with a 0-degree tip, a Kelman tip, or a flare tip. The flare is a modification of power intensity and the ABS of flow modification. In the ABS system, a 0.175-mm hole in the shaft permits a variable flow of fluid into the needle, even during occlusion. Therefore, occlusion is never allowed to occur (Figure 1-7). This flow adjustment serves to minimize surge.

Vacuum Sources

There are 3 categories of vacuum sources or pumps. These are flow pumps, vacuum pumps, and hybrid pumps.

1. The primary example of the flow pump type is the peristaltic pump. These pumps allow for independent control of both aspiration rate (flow) and aspiration level (vacuum).

2. The primary example of the vacuum pump is the venturi pump. This pump type allows direct control of only vacuum level. Flow is dependent upon vacuum level setting. Additional examples are the rotary vane and diaphragmatic pumps.

3. The primary example of the hybrid pump is Abbott Medical Optics' (Santa Ana, CA) Sovereign peristaltic pump or the Bausch & Lomb (Aliso Viejo, CA) Concentrix pump. These pumps are interesting because they are able to act like either a vacuum or flow pump dependent upon programming. They are the most recent supplement to pump types. They are generally controlled by digital inputs, creating incredible flexibility and responsiveness. They are rapidly becoming the standard type of pump for modern phaco.

The challenge to the surgeon is to balance the effect of phaco intensity (which tends to push nuclear fragments off of the phaco tip) with the effect of flow (which attracts fragments toward the phaco tip) and vacuum (which holds the fragments on the phaco tip). Generally, low flow slows down intraocular events, and high vacuum speeds them up. Low or zero vacuum is helpful while sculpting a hard or large nucleus, where the high-power intensity of the tip may be applied near the iris or anterior capsule. Zero vacuum will prevent inadvertent aspiration of the iris or capsule, preventing significant morbidity.

Surge

A principal limiting factor in the selection of high levels of vacuum or flow is the development of surge. When the phaco tip is occluded, flow is interrupted and vacuum builds to its preset level (Figure 1-8). Emulsification of the occluding fragment then clears the occlusion. Flow immediately begins at the preset level in the presence of the high vacuum level. In addition, if the aspiration line tubing is not reinforced to prevent collapse (tubing compliance), the tubing will have constricted during the occlusion. It then expands on occlusion break. The expansion is an additional source of vacuum production. These factors cause a rush of fluid from the anterior segment into the phaco tip. The fluid in the AC may not be replaced rapidly enough by infusion to prevent shallowing of the anterior chamber. Therefore, there is subsequent rapid anterior movement of the posterior capsule.

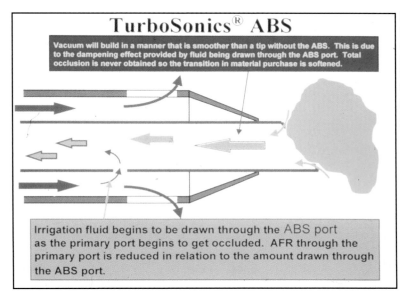

Figure 1-7. A 0.175-mm hole drilled in the shaft of the ABS tip provides an alternate path for fluid to flow into the needle when there is an occlusion at the phaco tip. (Reprinted with permission from Alcon, Fort Worth, TX.)

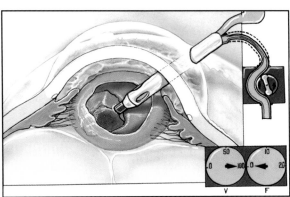

Figure 1-8. Occlusion: vacuum builds, flow falls toward zero, tubing collapses. (Reprinted with permission from Fishkind WJ. *Complications in Phacoemulsification*. New York, NY: Thieme Medical Publishers; 2002.)

This abrupt forceful stretching of the bag around nuclear fragments may be a cause of capsular tears. In addition, the posterior capsule can be literally sucked into the phaco tip, tearing it. The magnitude of the surge is contingent on the presurge settings of flow and vacuum (Figure 1-9). Surge is therefore modified by selecting lower levels of flow and vacuum.[5]

PHACO CHOP

Phaco chop requires no sculpting. Therefore, the procedure is initiated with high vacuum and flow and linear pulsed phaco power. For a 0-degree tip, when emulsifying a hard nucleus, a small trough may be required to create adequate room for the phaco tip to burrow deep into the nucleus. For a 15-degree or a 30-degree tip, the tip should be rotated bevel down to engage the nucleus. The phaco tip should be buried into the endonucleus with the minimal amount of power necessary. If the phaco tip is inserted into the nucleus with excess power, the adjacent nucleus will be emulsified, creating a poor seal between nucleus and tip. This will make it impossible to remove fragments because the tip will just "let go" of the nuclear material (Figure 1-10). Additionally, the bevel should be turned toward the fragment to create a seal between tip and fragment, allowing a vacuum to build and create holding power (Figure 1-11).

Figure 1-9. Occlusion break: vacuum drops to zero. Flow rapidly increases to preset. Tubing expands. Outflow exceeds inflow. Anterior chamber begins to shallow. (Reprinted with permission from Fishkind WJ. *Complications in Phacoemulsification*. New York, NY: Thieme Medical Publishers; 2002.)

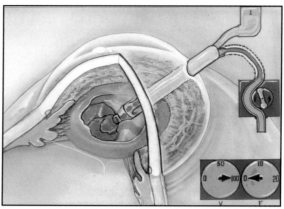

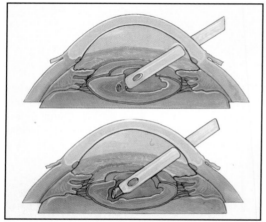

Figure 1-10. Top: power adequate to enter nucleus but maintain seal between the tip and nucleus. This will allow the tip to maneuver the nucleus. Bottom: excessive power causes the nucleus around the tip to be emulsified. There is no seal around the phaco tip. The nucleus cannot be maneuvered by the tip. (Reprinted with permission from Fishkind WJ. *Complications in Phacoemulsification*. New York, NY: Thieme Medical Publishers; 2002.)

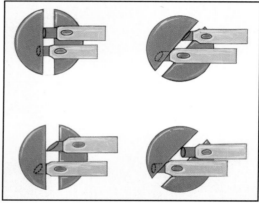

Figure 1-11. Top: correct position of nucleus in relation to the phaco tip. Occlusion is effortless. Bottom: incorrect orientation. Occlusion is difficult. (Reprinted with permission from Fishkind WJ. *Complications in Phacoemulsification*. New York, NY: Thieme Medical Publishers; 2002.)

HORIZONTAL CHOP

A few bursts or pulses of phaco energy will allow the tip to be buried within the nucleus. It then can be drawn toward the incision to allow the chopper access to the epi-endo nuclear junction. If the nucleus comes off of the phaco tip, excessive power has produced a space around the tip, impeding vacuum holding power as noted above. The first chop is then produced (Figure 1-12). Minimal rotation of the nucleus will allow for creation of the second chop. The first pie-shaped segment of nucleus is mobilized with high vacuum and elevated to the iris plane. There it is emulsified with low linear power, high vacuum, and moderate flow. The process of chopping and segment removal is continued until the endonucleus is removed.

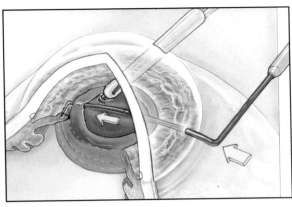

Figure 1-12. Horizontal chop. The phaco tip is drawn toward the wound and the chopper is placed into the epinucleus-endonucleus junctions, often under the anterior capsule. (Reprinted with permission from Fishkind WJ. *Complications in Phacoemulsification.* New York, NY: Thieme Medical Publishers; 2002.)

VERTICAL CHOP

Once the phaco tip is embedded within the nucleus, a sharp chopper (Nichamin HydroChopper, Katena, Denville, NJ) is pushed down into the mass of the nucleus at the same time the phaco tip is elevated (Figure 1-13). The chopper is then advanced down and left and the phaco tip up and right. This creates a cleavage in the nucleus. The process is repeated until the entire nucleus is chopped. The segments created are then elevated to the plane of the pupil and emulsified.

VITRECTOMY

Most phaco machines are equipped with a vitreous cutter that is activated by compressed air or by an electric motor. As noted previously, preservation of a deep anterior chamber is dependent upon a balance of inflow and outflow. For vitrectomy, a 23-gauge cannula or chamber maintainer inserted through a paracentesis provides inflow. Bottle height should be adequate to prevent chamber collapse. The vitrector should be inserted through another paracentesis. If equipped with a Charles sleeve, this should be removed and discarded. Utilizing a flow of 20 cc/min, vacuum of 250 mm Hg, and a cutting rate of 250 to 350 cuts/min, the vitrector should be placed through the tear in the posterior capsule, orifice facing upward, pulling vitreous out of the anterior chamber. The vitreous should be removed to the level of the posterior capsule (Figure 1-14).

Alternatively, the vitrector can be inserted through a pars plana incision 3 mm posterior to the limbus. In an effort to better visualize the vitreous for thorough vitrectomy, unpreserved sterile prednisone acetate (Kenalog) can be injected into the vitreous. The prednisone particles adhere to the vitreous strands, making the invisible visible.

MICROINCISIONAL CATARACT SURGERY

Surgeons inevitably aspire to construct smaller incisions. Recently, due to the use of thin-walled phaco needles and thin infusion sleeves, it is possible to create incisions 2.0 mm or smaller. Any incision smaller than 2.0 mm is classified as microincisional.

BIMANUAL MICROINCISION CATARACT SURGERY

The development of micropulse, "cold phaco" has led to the performance of phaco with an unsleeved tip. This allows for two 20-gauge, 1.4-mm incisions or 21-gauge, 1.2-mm incisions. The instrumentation for this procedure is important and the relationship between the instrument and incision size is essential. If there is too tight a wound, it is

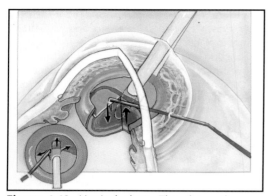

Figure 1-13. Vertical chop. The sharp chopper is placed adjacent to the phaco tip and plunged into the substance of the endonucleus. (Reprinted with permission from Fishkind WJ. *Complications in Phacoemulsification*. New York, NY: Thieme Medical Publishers; 2002.)

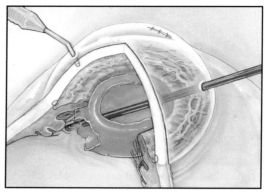

Figure 1-14. The vitrector is placed through a new paracentesis deep to the rent in the posterior capsule. Irrigation is via a cannula. (Reprinted with permission from Fishkind WJ. *Complications in Phacoemulsification*. New York, NY: Thieme Medical Publishers; 2002.)

difficult to manipulate the instruments. If the wound is too large, excessive outflow permits chamber shallowing. Microincision phaco is reportedly more efficient than standard because the flow from the irrigating chopper in the direction of the phaco tip captures fragments and carries them toward the phaco tip. The small incisions cause less disruption of the blood aqueous barrier and are more stable and secure. With insertion of an intraocular lens through the 1.4-mm incision, there is less disruption of ocular integrity with immediate return to full activities and less risk of postoperative wound complications.

COAXIAL MICROINCISIONAL CATARACT SURGERY

Stellaris (Bausch & Lomb) has pioneered a thin-walled phaco tip and sleeve combination that can be used to perform phaco through a 1.8-mm incision. The effectiveness of the procedure is unexpected in that despite the small incision size, the anterior chamber remains deep and stable, making the learning curve minimal.

MICROPHAKONIT

The microphakonit procedure (700-μm cataract surgery) was conceived by Dr. Amar Agarwal. This is at present the smallest incision by which a cataract can be removed, creating a sub-1-mm incision. In this procedure, the incisions are prepared with a purpose-designed Agarwal 0.8-mm microphakonit knife (MicroSurgical Technology, Redmond, WA). A microphakonit 700-μm needle and 700-μm irrigating chopper (both MicroSurgical Technology) are then used to perform phacoemulsification. A microfiltered gas-forced infusion, produced with the aid of a simple fish-aquarium air pump, provides forced infusion. Bimanual irrigation and aspiration is then performed with a 700-μm bimanual irrigation and aspiration set (MicroSurgical Technology).[6]

SUMMARY

It has been said that the phaco procedure is a blend of technology and technique. Awareness of the principles that influence phaco machine settings is requisite for the performance of a proficient and safe operation. Additionally, during the procedure, there is often a demand for modifying the initial parameters. A thorough understanding of fundamental principles will enhance the capability of the surgeon to appropriately respond to this requirement. It is a fundamental principle that, through relentless evaluation of the interaction of the machine and the phaco technique, the skillful surgeon will find innovative methods to enhance the technique.

References

1. Buratto L, Osher RH, Masket S, eds. *Cataract Surgery in Complicated Cases*. Thorofare, NJ: SLACK Incorporated; 2000.
2. Fishkind WJ, ed. *Complications in Phacoemulsification: Recognition, Avoidance, and Management*. New York, NY: Thieme; 2002.
3. Fishkind WJ. Pop goes the microbubbles. ESCRS Film Festival Grand Prize Winner; 1998.
4. Fishkind WJ, Neuhann TF, Steinert RF. The phaco machine. In: Steinert RF, ed. *Cataract Surgery: Technique, Complications and Management*. 2nd ed. Philadelphia, PA: WB Saunders; 2004:61-77.
5. Seibel BS. *Phacodynamics: Mastering the Tools and Techniques of Phacoemulsification Surgery*. 3rd ed. Thorofare, NJ: SLACK Incorporated; 1999.
6. Agarwal A, Kumar DA, Jacob S, Agarwal A. In vivo analysis of wound architecture in 700 µm microphakonit cataract surgery. *Cataract Refract Surg.* 2008;34:1554-1560.

CHAPTER 2

Wound Architecture, Induced Astigmatism, and Aberrations in MICS and In Vivo Analysis of 700-μm Cataract Surgery

Dhivya Ashok Kumar, MD; Gaurav Prakash, MS; Vidya Nair, MD; and Amar Agarwal, MS, FRCS, FRCOphth

The advances in phacoemulsification techniques and phacomachines along with the invention of foldable intraocular lenses (IOLs) made clear corneal incisions (CCIs) of less than 3 mm possible.[1-13] The current objective or goal in cataract surgery is to achieve the preferred visual outcome with minimal trauma to the cornea. Microincisional cataract surgery (MICS) continues to gain more attention because of less postoperative-induced astigmatism compared to conventional phacoemulsification. With the introduction of high-speed anterior segment optical coherence tomography (OCT), it is now possible to visualize the wound morphology.[14-16]

Wound Evaluation

We looked for evidence of endothelial misalignment, epithelial misalignment, coaptation loss, stromal hydration, and Descemet's status in the wound site with anterior segment OCT.

Twelve eyes of 11 patients were included in the study. Twenty-four clear corneal wounds (the main port and the side port) were studied and included. Twelve eyes of 11 patients underwent phacoemulsification with Agarwal's 700-μm phaco tip (MicroSurgical Technology, Redmond, WA; Figure 2-1). Five out of 12 eyes had no IOL implantation and 7 eyes underwent foldable IOL implantation by extension of the main port of the microphakonit incision with a 2.8-mm keratome. The incisions were examined in the immediate postoperative period with mean duration of 30 minutes from the surgery, followed by day 1, day 3, and day 7 postoperative periods. Out of 24 clear corneal wounds, 17 were microphakonit without extension.

Microphakonit With No Wound Extension

ENDOTHELIAL AND EPITHELIAL MISALIGNMENT

Microphakonit wounds showed good endothelial alignment by day 3 (Figure 2-2). On comparing the correlation (Table 2-1) between the change in the endothelial alignment and stromal hydration from immediate postoperative time to day 7 in microphakonit, there was no significant correlation seen. There was a positive correlation ($r = 0.811$, $P = 0.002$) between the incision angle and endothelial misalignment (Figure 2-3). No fish mouthing or epithelial misalignment was seen in any of the microphakonit incisions.

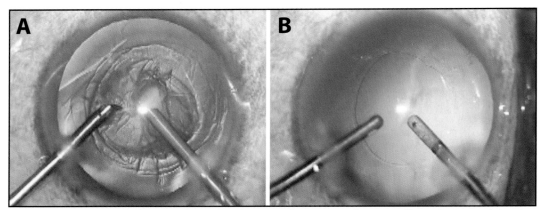

Figure 2-1. (A) Microphakonit performed with Agarwal's 700-μm phaco needle and 700-μm irrigating chopper (MicroSurgical Technology). (B) Bimanual irrigation aspiration done with 700-μm bimanual irrigation and aspiration set (MicroSurgical Technology). (Photo courtesy of Dr. Agarwal's Group of Eye Hospitals and Eye Research Centre, Chennai, India.)

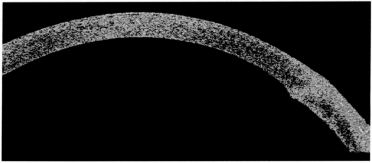

Figure 2-2. Anterior segment optical coherence tomography cross-sectional image of the microphakonit wound showing good endothelial alignment on day 3. (Photo courtesy of Dr. Agarwal's Group of Eye Hospitals and Eye Research Centre, Chennai, India.)

Table 2-1

CORRELATION ANALYSIS*

	Immediate–Day 1		Day 1–Day 3		Day 3–Day 7	
	r-Value	p-Value	r-Value	p-Value	r-Value	p-Value
EN-SH	0.098	0.707	-0.101	0.699	-0.162	0.534
EN-CL	-0.076	0.771	-0.187	0.471	-0.319	0.211
SH-CL	0.883	0.000	0.883	0.000	0.881	0.000
IOP-CL	—	—	—	—	-0.604	0.01
IOP-EN	—	—	-0.321	0.208	-0.347	0.172

*EN indicates endothelial misalignment; SH, stromal hydration; CL, coaptation loss; IOP, intraocular pressure; r, Pearson's correlation coefficient.

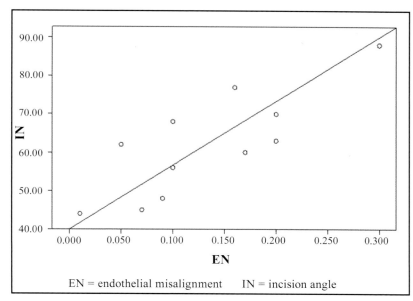

Figure 2-3. Scatterplot showing the correlation of endothelial misalignment and incision angle. (Photo courtesy of Dr. Agarwal's Group of Eye Hospitals and Eye Research Centre, Chennai, India.)

EN = endothelial misalignment   IN = incision angle

COAPTATION LOSS

The mean coaptation loss seen in microphakonit was 0.03 ± 0.06 mm in the immediate postoperative period. Twelve out of the 17 incisions (70.5%) showed no coaptation loss in the immediate postoperative period. Dense wound apposition line was seen as early as day 1 (Figure 2-4) in all eyes with microphakonit. There was a significant positive correlation (Figure 2-5) seen between the change in stromal hydration and coaptation loss in the postoperative period (see Table 2-1).

STROMAL HYDRATION

The mean immediate postoperative stromal hydration in microphakonit wound was 1.08 ± 0.23 mm. The resolution of stromal hydration was seen by the change in the peripheral corneal thickness.

MICROPHAKONIT WITH 2.8-MM WOUND EXTENSION

On comparison of microphakonit with 2.8-mm extension (Table 2-2) in the 7 eyes that underwent IOL implantation, there was no significant difference in the mean early (within 30 minutes of surgery) endothelial misalignment ($P = 0.253$) and coaptation loss ($P = 0.535$) between the microphakonit with and without 2.8-mm extension: 29.4% of the 17 microphakonit incisions had coaptation loss in the immediate 30-minute postoperative period OCT, whereas 42.8% of the 2.8-mm incisions showed immediate coaptation loss. One out of 7 incisions of 2.8-mm extension had localized Descemet detachment seen in OCT and localized subclinical Descemet's tear was noted in 1 out of 17 of the microphakonit wounds.

CORRELATION OF INTRAOCULAR PRESSURE WITH WOUND ARCHITECTURE

The effect of intraocular pressure (IOP) was equal on both wounds (side or main port) in the same eye. There was no significant difference between the mean IOP of the eyes with and without endothelial misalignment ($P = 0.557$) or coaptation loss ($P = 0.237$) in the

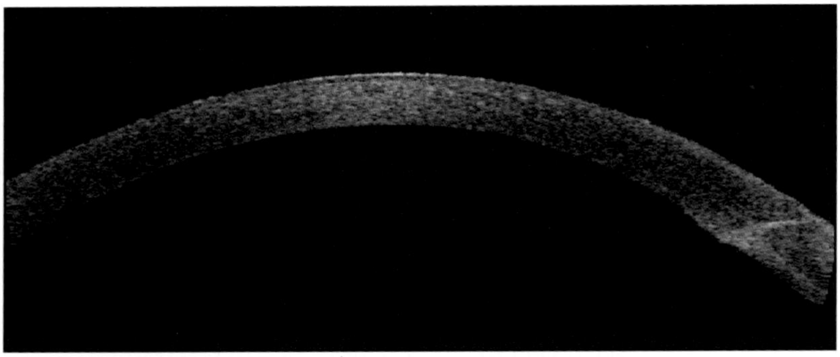

Figure 2-4. High-resolution cross-sectional image of the anterior segment optical coherence tomography showing dense apposition line in microphakonit wound. (Photo courtesy of Dr. Agarwal's Group of Eye Hospitals and Eye Research Centre, Chennai, India.)

Figure 2-5. Scatterplot showing the positive correlation between change in stromal hydration and coaptation loss in the postoperative period. (Photo courtesy of Dr. Agarwal's Group of Eye Hospitals and Eye Research Centre, Chennai, India.)

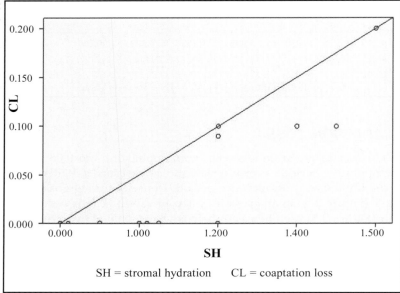

SH = stromal hydration   CL = coaptation loss

Table 2-2

MICROPHAKONIT WITH 2.8-MM EXTENSION*

	Endothelial Misalignment				Coaptation Loss			
Wound	Imm	Day 1	Day 3	Day 7	Imm	Day 1	Day 3	Day 7
1	0	0	0	0	0.07	0.05	0	0
2	0	0	0	0	0.1	0.09	0.09	0.04
3	0.2	0.15	0	0	0	0	0	0
4	0.02	0	0	0	0	0	0	0
5	0.18	0.2	0.1	0.08	0.07	0.07	0.06	0.06
6	0.1	0.2	0.16	0.17	0	0	0	0
7	0.4	0.34	0.3	0.2	0	0	0	0
Mean	0.128	0.127	0.08	0.064	0.034	0.03	0.021	0.014
SD	0.145	0.132	0.116	0.088	0.043	0.039	0.037	0.025

*Imm indicates immediate; SD, standard deviation.

17 microphakonit wounds. On comparing the endothelial misalignment in the 17 microphakonit wounds according to day 1 IOP, less than 10 mm Hg and more than 10 mm Hg, no significant difference was seen in the mean endothelial misalignment ($P = 0.857$) and coaptation loss ($P = 0.291$).

Corneal Topographic Changes

Orbscan (Bausch & Lomb, Aliso Viejo, CA) topography evaluation in a group of 9 eyes (Table 2-3) that underwent 700-µm cataract surgery without extension showed no significant postoperative changes (Figure 2-6). Incisions in which ThinOptX rollable IOL (Abingdon, VA) was implanted showed no change in corneal topography over the time period (Figures 2-7 and 2-8). In a study of postoperative-induced astigmatism after phakonit surgery (Table 2-4), topographical analysis showed a mean 0.98 ± 0.62 D (range 0.5 to 1.8 D) preoperatively and 1.1 ± 0.61 D (range 0.6 to 1.9 D) on postoperative day 1. The mean astigmatism at 3 months (Figure 2-9) postoperative was 1.02 ± 0.64 D. The topographic changes in eyes with 1.8-mm incision size and foldable IOL (Akreos MI60 IOL, Bausch & Lomb) implantation (Figure 2-10) have also been evaluated.

Induced astigmatism was significantly less in temporal corneal MICS than in small incision cataract surgery (SICS).[17] Focal wound-related flattening of the peripheral cornea and corneal surface irregularity were observed to be less after coaxial MICS (2 mm) than after SICS (2.65 mm) according to Hayashi et al.[18]

Table 2-3

ANALYSIS OF POSTOPERATIVE ASTIGMATISM IN MICROPHAKONIT*

	N	Mean	Std. Deviation	Minimum	Maximum
Preoperative	8	2.3938	1.43712	0.5	4.4
Postoperative	8	1.3625	0.84124	0.5	3.2

*N indicates number of eyes.

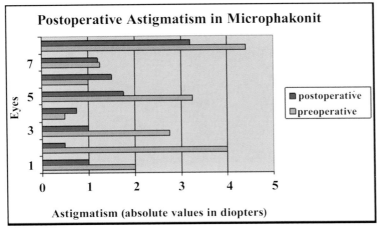

Figure 2-6. Bar diagram showing the postoperative astigmatism in eyes with microphakonit surgery. No significant change was observed ($p = 0.069$). (Photo courtesy of Dr. Agarwal's Group of Eye Hospitals and Eye Research Centre, Chennai, India.)

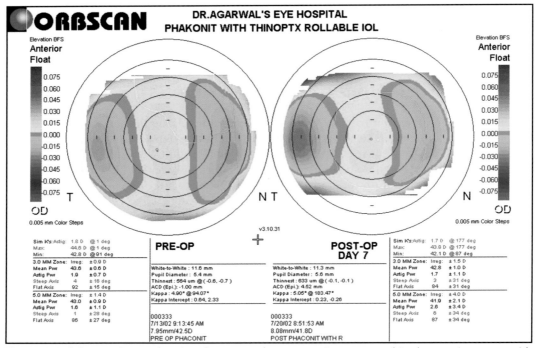

Figure 2-7. Orbscan picture showing the pre- and postoperative topographic changes in an eye with phakonit with ThinOptX rollable intraocular lens. (Photo courtesy of Dr. Agarwal's Group of Eye Hospitals and Eye Research Centre, Chennai, India.)

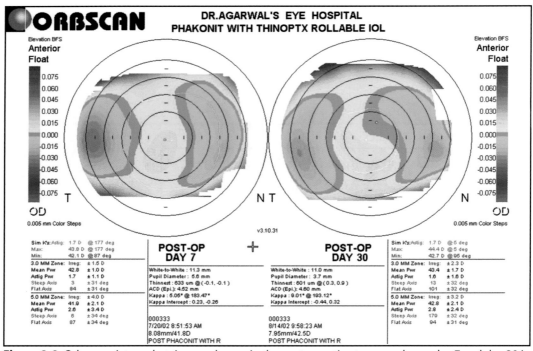

Figure 2-8. Orbscan picture showing no change in the postoperative topography on day 7 and day 30 in an eye with phakonit with ThinOptX rollable intraocular lens. (Photo courtesy of Dr. Agarwal's Group of Eye Hospitals and Eye Research Centre, Chennai, India.)

Table 2-4

ANALYSIS OF ASTIGMATISM IN PHAKONIT OVER A TIME PERIOD*

	N	Mean	Std. Deviation	Minimum	Maximum
Preoperative	5	0.98	0.62	0.5	1.8
POD 1	5	1.1	0.61	0.6	1.9
POD 7	5	1.12	0.58	0.5	1.7
POD 30	5	1.08	0.62	0.5	1.8
POD 90	5	1.02	0.64	0.3	1.7

*N indicates number of eyes; POD, postoperative day.

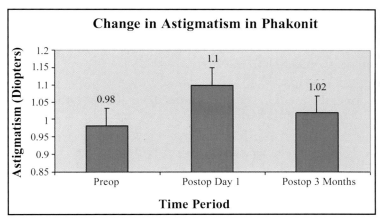

Figure 2-9. Error bar plot comparing the mean astigmatism in phakonit. (Photo courtesy of Dr. Agarwal's Group of Eye Hospitals and Eye Research Centre, Chennai, India.)

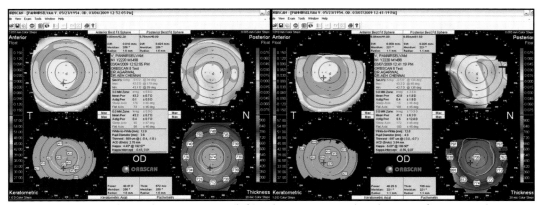

Figure 2-10. Pre- (right) and postoperative (left) Orbscan topographic changes of an eye with 1.8-mm clear corneal incision with foldable intraocular lens (Akreos MI60 IOL) implantation. (Photo courtesy of Dr. Agarwal's Group of Eye Hospitals and Eye Research Centre, Chennai, India.)

Corneal Aberrations Profile

Denoyer et al[19] compared 1.7-mm CCI in one eye with bimanual MICS (B-MICS) with 2.8-mm CCI of coaxial SICS in the other eye and concluded that biaxial MICS could improve the optical performances of the pseudophakic eye, reducing surgically induced corneal higher-order aberrations. Surgically induced corneal trefoil was significantly reduced in B-MICS eyes. MICS IOLs showed excellent modulation transfer function performance equal to conventional phacoemulsification IOLs by Optical Quality Analysis System (OQAS, Visiometrics, Terrassa, Spain) for a 5-mm pupil according to Alio et al.[20]

Advantages of Microincision

* *Faster wound healing*: The wound healing seemed to be faster in microphakonit without extension (Figure 2-11); 82.3% of the eyes had no endothelial gape on day 3 and 100% on day 7 (Figure 2-12) compared to 57.1% on day 3 and 57.1% on day 7 in 2.8-mm extended wounds.

* *No difference in healing in main or side port*: On comparing the main port with side port incision in the immediate postoperative period of the 5 eyes with microphakonit without IOL implantation, no significant difference in the wound morphology (namely coaptation loss [$P = 0.374$] and endothelial misalignment [$P = 0.146$]) was seen between the wounds with and without phaco needle.

* *Early tight closure at the incision site*: One of the advantages seen with microphakonit was that there was tight closure at the incision site in the immediate postoperative period (Figure 2-13) compared to the incisions in which extension was made.

* *Less fluid ingress and infection*: Tight closure at the incision site in the immediate postoperative period decreases the chance of ingress of fluid and organisms from the ocular surface into the anterior chamber and in turn decreases the chances of endophthalmitis.

* *Self-sealed/no sutures*: The incisions in microphakonit were also self-sealed without any suture and no external wound gaping as early as day 1, which was seen as a well-formed tunnel in OCT. Moreover, the incisions used for microphakonit[4-6] are so small and self-sealing that the chance of their opening as a result of lid or ocular movements is negligible.

* *Less postoperative leakage and shallow anterior chamber*: Microphakonit wounds have less postoperative leakage and a shallow anterior chamber; in addition, due to the properties of early wound apposition and healing, there is also a lesser incidence of postoperative infection.

* *No change with IOP*: There was no significant difference between the mean IOP of the eyes with and without endothelial misalignment or coaptation loss.

Summary

Corneal wound construction and design play a pivotal role in the prevention of postoperative inflammation and infection. A smaller incision results in less induced astigmatism, faster visual rehabilitation, and improved wound healing.

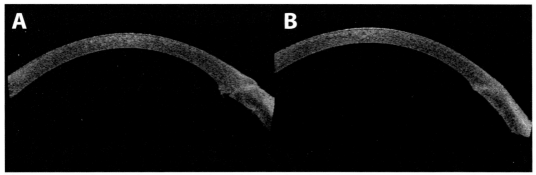

Figure 2-11. High-resolution cross-sectional image taken in the anterior segment optical coherence tomography showing wound healing over a period of time in microphakonit. (A) Immediately postoperative (30 min after surgery) shows endothelial misalignment. (B) Day 1 shows well-formed apposition line with decrease in endothelial misalignment. (Photo courtesy of Dr. Agarwal's Group of Eye Hospitals and Eye Research Centre, Chennai, India.)

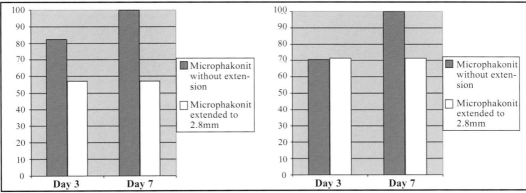

Figure 2-12. Graphical representation comparing wound healing in microphakonit wound without and with 2.8-mm extension. The left shows the percentage of wounds showing no endothelial misalignment. The right shows the percentage of wounds showing no coaptation loss. (Photo courtesy of Dr. Agarwal's Group of Eye Hospitals and Eye Research Centre, Chennai, India.)

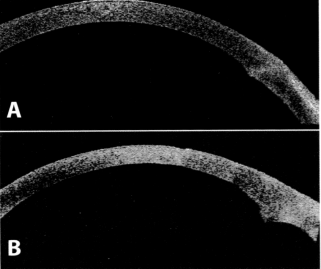

Figure 2-13. High-resolution cross-sectional image of wound in the anterior segment optical coherence tomography on day 1. (A) Microphakonit without extension. (B) Microphakonit with 2.8-mm extension. (Photo courtesy of Dr. Agarwal's Group of Eye Hospitals and Eye Research Centre, Chennai, India.)

REFERENCES

1. Agarwal A, Agarwal S, Agarwal A, Narang P, Narang S. Phakonit: phacoemulsification through a 0.9 mm incision. *J Cataract Refract Surg.* 2001;27(10):1548-1552.
2. Pandey S, Werner L, Agarwal A, et al. Phakonit: cataract removal through a sub 1.0 mm incision with implantation of the ThinOptX rollable IOL. *J Cataract Refract Surg.* 2002;28(9):1710-1713.
3. Agarwal A, Agarwal S, Agarwal A. Phakonit with an AcriTec IOL. *J Cataract Refract Surg.* 2003;29(4):854-855.
4. Agarwal A, Trivedi RH, Jacob S, Agarwal A, Agarwal S. Microphakonit: 700 micron cataract surgery. *Clin Ophthalmol.* 2007;1(3):323-325.
5. Agarwal A, Jacob S, Sinha S, Agarwal A. Combating endophthalmitis with microphakonit and no-anesthesia technique. *J Cataract Refract Surg.* 2007;33(12):2009-2011.
6. Agarwal A, Jacob S, Agarwal A. Combined microphakonit and 25-gauge transconjunctival sutureless vitrectomy. *J Cataract Refract Surg.* 2007;33(11):1839-1840.
7. Tsuneoka H, Shiba T, Takahashi Y. Feasibility of ultrasound cataract surgery with a 1.4 mm incision. *J Cataract Refract Surg.* 2001;27(6):934-940.
8. Tsuneoka H, Shiba T, Takahashi Y. Ultrasonic phacoemulsification using a 1.4 mm incision: clinical results. *J Cataract Refract Surg.* 2002;28(1):81-86.
9. Alió J, Rodríguez-Prats JL, Galal A, Ramzy M. Outcomes of microincision cataract surgery versus coaxial phacoemulsification. *Ophthalmology.* 2005;112(11):1997-2003.
10. Dosso AA, Cottet L, Burgener N, Di Nardo S. Outcomes of coaxial microincision cataract surgery versus conventional coaxial cataract surgery. *J Cataract Refract Surg.* 2008;34(2):284-288.
11. Agarwal A, Agarwal S, Agarwal A. Antichamber collapser. *J Cataract Refract Surg.* 2002;28(7):1085-1086.
12. Agarwal A, Agarwal S, Agarwal A. Phakonit: A new technique of removing cataracts through a 0.9 mm incision. In: Agarwal A, Agarwal S, Agarwal A, eds. *Phacoemulsification, Laser Cataract Surgery and Foldable IOLs*. New Delhi, India: Jaypee; 1998:139-143.
13. Agarwal A, Agarwal S, Agarwal A. Phakonit and laser phakonit: Lens surgery through a 0.9 mm incision. In: Agarwal A, Agarwal S, Agarwal A, eds. *Phacoemulsification, Laser Cataract Surgery and Foldable IOLs*. 2nd ed. New Delhi, India: Jaypee; 2000:204-216.
14. Calladine D, Packard R. Clear corneal incision architecture in the immediate postoperative period evaluated using optical coherence tomography. *J Cataract Refract Surg.* 2007;33(8):1429-1435.
15. Pandey SK, Werner L, Apple DJ, Agarwal A, Agarwal A, Agarwal S. No-anesthesia clear corneal phacoemulsification versus topical and topical plus intracameral anaesthesia: randomized clinical trial. *J Cataract Refract Surg.* 2001;27(10):1643-1650.
16. Agarwal A, Kumar DA, Jacob S, Agarwal A. In vivo analysis of wound architecture in 700 micron microphakonit surgery. *J Cataract Refract Surg.* 2008;34(9):1554-1560.
17. Tagawa K, Higashide T, Sugiyama K, Kawasaki K. Surgically induced astigmatism after micro and small clear temporal corneal incision in cataract surgery. *Nippon Ganka Gakkai Zasshi.* 2007;111(9):716-721.
18. Hayashi K, Yoshida M, Hayashi H. Postoperative corneal shape changes: microincision versus small-incision coaxial cataract surgery. *J Cataract Refract Surg.* 2009;35(2):233-239.
19. Denoyer A, Denoyer L, Marotte D, Georget M, Pisella PJ. Intraindividual comparative study of corneal and ocular wavefront aberrations after biaxial microincision versus coaxial small-incision cataract surgery. *Br J Ophthalmol.* 2008;92:1679-1684.
20. Alió JL, Schimchak P, Montés-Micó R, Galal A. Retinal image quality after microincision intraocular lens implantation. *J Cataract Refract Surg.* 2005;31(8):1557-1560.

CHAPTER 3

AIR PUMP, GAS-FORCED INFUSION, AND FLUIDICS

*Smita Narsimhan, FERC; Prashaant Chaudhry, MD;
Hiroshi Tsuneoka, MD; and Amar Agarwal, MS, FRCS, FRCOphth*

HISTORY

The main problem we had in bimanual microincisional cataract surgery (B-MICS)/phakonit was the destabilization of the anterior chamber during surgery. We solved it to a certain extent by using an 18-gauge irrigating chopper. Then Sunita Agarwal suggested the use of an antichamber collapser, which injects air into the infusion bottle (Figure 3-1). This pushes more fluid into the eye through the irrigating chopper and also prevents surge.[1-5] Thus, we were able to use a 20- or 21-gauge irrigating chopper, as well as solve the problem of destabilizing the anterior chamber during surgery. Now with microphakonit, because of gas-forced infusion, we are able to remove cataracts with a 0.7-mm irrigating chopper (22 gauge). Subsequently, we used this system in all of our coaxial phaco cases, including coaxial MICS (C-MICS), to prevent complications like posterior capsular ruptures and corneal damage.

Since the introduction of phacoemulsification by Kelman,[6] it has undergone revolutionary changes in an attempt to perfect the techniques of extracapsular cataract extraction surgery. Although advantageous in many aspects, this technique is not without its attending complications. A well-maintained anterior chamber without intraocular fluctuations is one of the prerequisites for safe phacoemulsification and phakonit.[7]

When an occluded fragment is held by high vacuum and then abruptly aspirated, fluid rushes into the phaco tip to equilibrate the built-up vacuum in the aspiration line, causing surge.[8] This leads to shallowing or collapse of the anterior chamber. Different machines employ a variety of methods to combat surge. These include usage of noncomplaint tubing, small bore aspiration line tubing, microflow tips, aspiration bypass systems, dual linear foot pedal control, and incorporation of sophisticated microprocessors to sense the anterior chamber pressure fluctuations.[9]

The surgeon-dependent variables to counteract surge include good wound construction with minimal leakage and selection of appropriate machine parameters depending on the stage of the surgery.[10] An anterior chamber maintainer has also been described in literature to prevent surge, but an extra side port makes it an inconvenient procedure.

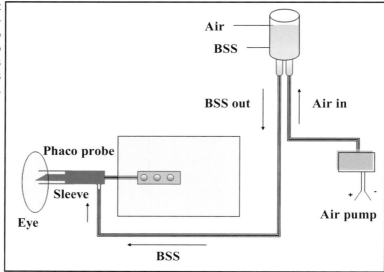

Figure 3-1. Diagrammatic representation of the connection of the air pump to the infusion bottle. (Photo courtesy of Dr. Agarwal's Group of Eye Hospitals and Eye Research Centre, Chennai, India.)

We started a simple and effective method to prevent anterior chamber collapse during phacoemulsification and phakonit in 1999 by increasing the velocity of the fluid inflow into the anterior chamber. This is achieved by an automated air pump that pumps atmospheric air through an air filter into the infusion bottle, thereby preventing surge. We stumbled upon this idea when we were operating cases with phakonit[1] when we wanted more fluid entering the eye, but now we also use it in all of our coaxial phaco cases.[2]

AIR PUMP

An automated air pump is used to push air into the infusion bottle, thus increasing the pressure with which fluid flows into the eye. This increases the steady-state pressure of the eye, keeping the anterior chamber deep and well maintained during the entire procedure. This makes phakonit and phacoemulsification a relatively safe procedure by reducing surge even at high vacuum levels.

TECHNIQUE

A locally manufactured automated device used in fish tanks (aquariums) to supply oxygen is utilized to forcefully pump air into the irrigation bottle. This pump is easily available in aquarium shops. It has an electromagnetic motor that moves a lever attached to a collapsible rubber cap. There is an inlet with a valve that sucks in atmospheric air as the cap expands. On collapsing, the valve closes and the air is pushed into an intravenous (IV) line connected to the infusion bottle (see Figure 3-1). The lever vibrates at a frequency of approximately 10 oscillations per second. The electromagnetic motor is weak enough to stop once the pressure in the closed system (ie, the anterior chamber) reaches about 50 mm Hg. The rubber cap ceases to expand at this pressure level. A switch in the air pump can also increase the pressure up to 100 mm Hg. A Millipore air filter (Billerica, MA) is used between the air pump and the infusion bottle so that the air pumped into the bottle is free from particulate matter.

METHOD

1. First, the balanced salt solution (BSS) bottle is placed on the IV stand.
2. An air pump (the same type that is used in aquariums to supply oxygen to fish) is plugged into an electrical socket.
3. An IV set now connects the air pump to the infusion bottle. The tubing passes from the air pump and the end of the tubing is inserted into the infusion bottle.
4. When the air pump is switched on, it pumps air into the infusion bottle. This air goes to the top of the bottle and, because of the pressure, it pumps the fluid down with greater force. With this, the fluid now flows from the infusion bottle to reach the phaco handpiece or irrigating chopper. The amount of fluid now coming out of the handpiece is greater than what would normally come out and has more force.
5. A Millipore air filter is connected between the air pump and the infusion bottle so that the air that is being pumped into the bottle is sterile.
6. This extra amount of fluid coming out compensates for the surge that would otherwise occur.

CONTINUOUS INFUSION

Before we enter the eye, we fill it with viscoelastic. Once the tip of the phaco handpiece (in phaco) or irrigating chopper (in phakonit) is inside the anterior chamber, we shift to continuous irrigation. This is helpful for surgeons who are just starting phaco or phakonit as well as the more accomplished surgeon. This way, the surgeon never comes to position 0 and the anterior chamber never collapses.

ADVANTAGES

1. With the air pump, the posterior capsule is pushed back and there is a deep anterior chamber.
2. The phenomenon of surge is neutralized. This prevents posterior capsular rupture.
3. Postoperative striate keratitis is reduced because there is a deep anterior chamber.
4. One can operate on hard cataracts quite comfortably because striate keratitis does not occur postoperatively.
5. The surgical time is shorter because one can emulsify the nuclear pieces much faster since surge does not occur.
6. One can comfortably do cases under topical or no anesthesia as the chamber does not shallow if the patient squeezes his or her eyes during surgery.
7. It is quite comfortable to do cases under topical or no anesthesia.

TOPICAL OR NO-ANESTHESIA CATARACT SURGERY

When one operates under topical or no anesthesia, the main problem is that sometimes the pressure is high, especially if the patient squeezes the eye. In such cases, the posterior capsule comes up anteriorly and one can produce a posterior capsular rupture. To solve this problem, surgeons tend to work more anteriorly, performing supracapsular phacoemulsification/phakonit. The disadvantage of this is that striate keratitis tends to occur.

With the air pump, this problem does not occur. When we use the air pump, the posterior capsule is pushed back as if we are operating on a patient under a block. In other words, there is a lot of space between the posterior capsule and the cornea, preventing striate keratitis and inadvertent posterior capsular rupture.

INTERNAL GAS-FORCED INFUSION

Internal gas-forced infusion was started by Arturo Pérez-Arteaga from Mexico. The anterior vented gas-forced infusion system (AVGFI) of the Accurus Surgical System (Alcon, Fort Worth, TX) is used. This is a system incorporated in the Accurus machine that creates a positive infusion pressure inside the eye; it was designed by the Alcon engineers to control the intraocular pressure (IOP) during posterior segment surgery. It consists of an air pump and a regulator inside the machine; the air is pushed inside the bottle of intraocular solution, and the fluid is actively pushed inside the eye without raising or lowering the bottle. The control of the air pump is digitally integrated in the Accurus panel; it also can be controlled via the remote. The footswitch can be preset with the minimum and maximum desired fluid inside the eye and it goes directly to this value with the simple touch of the footswitch. Arturo Pérez-Arteaga recommends presetting the infusion pump at 100 mm Hg; this is enough irrigation force to perform a microincision phaco. This parameter is preset in the panel and as the minimal irrigation force in the footswitch. He also recommends presetting the maximum irrigation force at 130 to 140 mm Hg in the foot pedal so if a surge occurs during the procedure, the surgeon can increase the irrigation force by a simple touch of the footswitch to the right. With the AVGFI, the surgeon has the capability to increase these values. A Millipore filter is used between the tubing and the air pump (Figure 3-2).

STELLARIS DIGIFLOW PRESSURIZED INFUSION

Bausch & Lomb (Aliso Viejo, CA) installed an air pump in their Stellaris machine in 2009 called the DigiFlow Pressurized Infusion. The advantage of this is that the air pump, which was an external gas-forced infusion system, is now inside the machine (Figure 3-3). Another advantage is that there is a monitor in the panel of the machine and one can lower or raise the pressure of the gas-forced infusion.

AIR PUMP–ASSISTED PHACO FOR MANAGING CASES WITH INCOMPLETE RHEXIS

The idea of this concept was given by Dr. Smita Narsimhan. In the event of a runaway capsulorrhexis, continuing with phacoemulsification carries the risk of extension of the capsular tear through the equator onto the posterior capsule. This can potentially lead to nucleus drop and vitreous loss and reduces the chance of a stable, in-the-bag intraocular lens (IOL) implantation. Multiple techniques can be used in the event of a tear. These include starting the capsulorrhexis from the opposite side to include the tear and backward traction on the base of the capsular flap, but these are not always successful. This technique may be used to complete phacoemulsification following an irretrievable anterior capsular tear with the assistance of an air pump (gas-forced infusion) in cataracts with nuclear sclerosis grade 1 to 3 or white cataracts in patients under 60 years of age.

The anterior capsulorrhexis is started as a capsular nick from the center, which is then moved to the right. The capsular flap is then lifted off and teased downward (Figure 3-4).

AIR PUMP, GAS-FORCED INFUSION, AND FLUIDICS

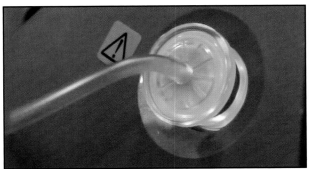

Figure 3-2. Millipore filter to connect the air pump to the tubing. Air pump in the Stellaris machine. (Photo courtesy of Dr. Agarwal's Group of Eye Hospitals and Eye Research Centre, Chennai, India.)

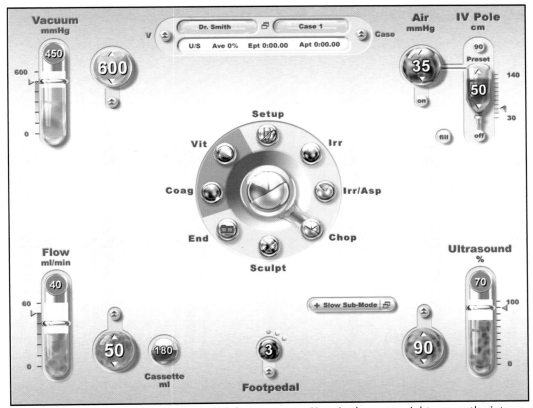

Figure 3-3. Stellaris DigiFlow pressurized infusion system. Note in the upper right corner the intravenous pole height in cm and next to it the air pump (gas-forced infusion pressure) in mm of mercury. (Photo courtesy of Dr. Agarwal's Group of Eye Hospitals and Eye Research Centre, Chennai, India.)

Because the maximum tendency to lose the capsulorrhexis is near its completion, we are usually left with an incomplete capsulorrhexis superiorly and to the right. Because all manipulations will be directed down and to the left, the chances of the capsulorrhexis extending will be less. For a left-handed surgeon, one should start from the center and move to the left. Following an irretrievable anterior capsular tear (Figure 3-5), we refrain from making further manipulations that may extend the tear to the posterior capsule. If there is suspicion of posterior capsular extension of the tear, we prefer to convert the surgery to an extracapsular cataract extraction (ECCE). The anterior capsule is then flattened with the help of viscoelastics, and we make a nick from the opposite side using a

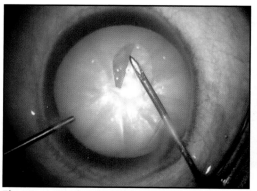 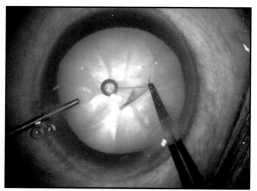

Figure 3-4. Rhexis started in a mature cataract. (Photo courtesy of Dr. Agarwal's Group of Eye Hospitals and Eye Research Centre, Chennai, India.)

Figure 3-5. Capsulorrhexis running away to the periphery. (Photo courtesy of Dr. Agarwal's Group of Eye Hospitals and Eye Research Centre, Chennai, India.)

cystitome or Vannas scissor (Appasamy Associates, Chennai, India) and complete the capsulorrhexis. The viscoelastic in the anterior chamber (AC) is then expressed out to make the globe hypotonous, following which a gentle hydrodissection (Figure 3-6) is done at a site 90 degrees from the tear while pressing the posterior lip of the incision to prevent any rise in IOP. No attempt is made to press on the center of the nucleus to complete the fluid wave. The fluid is usually sufficient to prolapse one pole of the nucleus out of the capsular bag (Figure 3-7); otherwise, it is removed by embedding the phacoemulsification probe, making sure not to exert any downward pressure and then gently pulling the nucleus anteriorly. The whole nucleus is brought out into the AC and no nuclear division techniques are tried in the bag.

Phacoemulsification can be started at this stage for cataracts with nuclear sclerosis grades 1 to 3, but it is safer to convert to an ECCE for nuclear sclerosis grade 4. Phacoemulsification is started with the gas-forced infusion in place and the bottle height 75 cm above eye level (Figure 3-8). The infusion is kept on continuous mode at all times. This prevents the AC from collapsing even if the surgeon takes his or her foot off of the machine. Because the entire nucleus is prolapsed into the anterior chamber and emulsified, this prevents any stretch on the torn capsulorrhexis. The gas-forced infusion provides for a deep anterior chamber, pushes the posterior capsule back, and prevents surge to allow safe anterior chamber phacoemulsification. While withdrawing the probe, viscoelastic is injected simultaneously through the side port incision. Irrigation aspiration is performed in Cap Vac mode with the aspiration set at 5 mm Hg, the flow rate at 6 mL/min, and the gas-forced infusion pump on (Figures 3-9 and 3-10). In the presence of a thick epinucleus, we first inject viscoelastic between the capsule and the cortical matter, 90 degrees from the site of the tear, to express the epinuclear plate into the anterior chamber. The epinucleus is then aspirated in the anterior chamber, keeping the vacuum at 120 mm Hg and flow rate at 20 mL/min. The cortex in the region of the capsular tear is aspirated out last. The anterior chamber and bag are partially filled with a viscoelastic and the IOL is injected, introducing the leading haptic into the bag but pointing away from the area of the tear and not directing the IOL too posteriorly (Figure 3-11). The IOL is gently manipulated into the capsular bag with the help of a Y rod (Agarwal's globe stabilization rod, Katena, Denville, NJ) giving a final orientation of the haptics 90 degrees away from the anterior capsular tear.

AIR PUMP, GAS-FORCED INFUSION, AND FLUIDICS

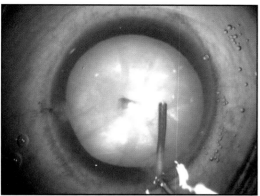

Figure 3-6. Hydrodissection done. (Photo courtesy of Dr. Agarwal's Group of Eye Hospitals and Eye Research Centre, Chennai, India.)

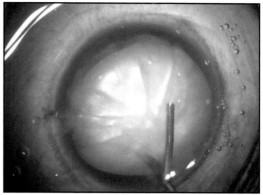

Figure 3-7. Nucleus prolapsed into the anterior chamber. (Photo courtesy of Dr. Agarwal's Group of Eye Hospitals and Eye Research Centre, Chennai, India.)

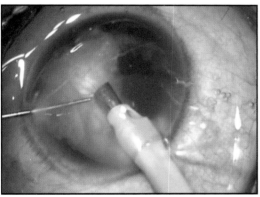

Figure 3-8. Nucleus being removed by phacoemulsification in the supracapsular area after prolapsing it into the anterior chamber. The air pump is used so no damage occurs to the corneal endothelium because the chamber is quite deep. (Photo courtesy of Dr. Agarwal's Group of Eye Hospitals and Eye Research Centre, Chennai, India.)

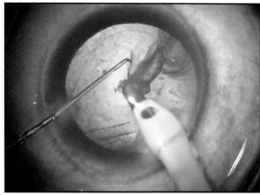

Figure 3-9. Irrigation aspiration being performed in the Cap Vac mode. (Photo courtesy of Dr. Agarwal's Group of Eye Hospitals and Eye Research Centre, Chennai, India.)

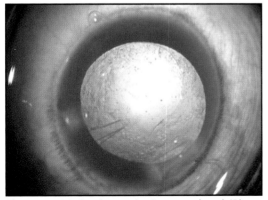

Figure 3-10. Irrigation aspiration completed. (Photo courtesy of Dr. Agarwal's Group of Eye Hospitals and Eye Research Centre, Chennai, India.)

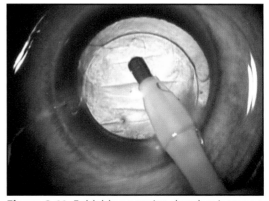

Figure 3-11. Foldable posterior chamber intraocular lens implanted. (Photo courtesy of Dr. Agarwal's Group of Eye Hospitals and Eye Research Centre, Chennai, India.)

CHAPTER 3

FLUIDICS

The advantages of B-MICS, however, are not limited to small incision size. There are also major differences in the intraocular fluidics of the infusion solution between these 2 techniques. In C-MICS (Figure 3-12), the phaco tip is equipped with an infusion sleeve, and infusion and aspiration are performed along the same axis. In contrast, B-MICS places the infusion and aspiration ports on separate instruments (Figure 3-13). This positioning results in unique fluidics for B-MICS and makes it possible to perform highly noninvasive surgery that is also safe.

FLUIDICS IN COAXIAL MICROINCISIONAL CATARACT SURGERY

With coaxial phaco, the aspiration port is positioned close to the infusion port, and the relative positioning of those 2 ports cannot be changed. In that situation, some of the infusion solution that flows out of the holes in the infusion sleeve never circulates within the eye but is immediately aspirated into the phaco tip (Figure 3-14A). This is called *shortcut flow* and requires the wasteful use of extra infusion solution that does not contribute to maintaining the stability of the anterior chamber depth.

In addition, the direction of flow of the infusion solution in coaxial phaco is opposite to the direction of aspiration of nuclear fragments. As a result, the infusion solution tends to push the nuclear fragments away from the aspiration port (Figure 3-14B). In order to counter the effects of this flow, it is necessary to increase the aspiration pressure.

Coaxial phaco requires elevated aspiration pressure in order to increase aspiration efficiency. However, higher aspiration pressure is associated with increased risk of surge, which is prevented by elevating the infusion bottle. The resulting increase in infusion pressure causes a stronger flow of infusion solution against the nuclear fragments. This becomes a vicious circle, necessitating substantial increases in aspiration pressure and infusion pressure in order to improve aspiration efficiency.

When surgery is performed under conditions such as these, the intraocular pressure can fluctuate considerably during the procedure, and the invasiveness of the surgery is greatly increased. In addition, because the aspiration port is generally positioned below the infusion port on the phaco tip, it is easy to accidentally aspirate the posterior capsule when the phaco tip is pointed downward and the aspiration pressure is increased.

FLUIDICS IN BIMANUAL MICROINCISIONAL CATARACT SURGERY

With B-MICS, the infusion port is separated from the aspiration port, and the positional relationship of these 2 ports can be freely changed. Because the aspiration port and the infusion port are separated, no shortcut flow develops, and the infusion solution can be used to push nuclear fragments toward the aspiration port (Figure 3-15). This makes it possible to efficiently aspirate the nuclear fragments at aspiration pressures lower than those required for coaxial phaco.

B-MICS surgery is characterized by good aspiration efficiency even at low settings for infusion pressure and aspiration pressure. As phacoemulsification and aspiration of the nucleus is performed efficiently while maintaining nonturbulent conditions in the anterior chamber, there is little variation in IOP during the procedure, and the surgery becomes highly noninvasive.

In contrast, when high aspiration settings are selected to increase aspiration efficiency, it becomes necessary to elevate the infusion bottle. This point should be noted because the higher infusion pressure can cause small fragments of nucleus within the anterior chamber to collect around the phaco tip at the insertion site, which reduces aspiration efficiency.

AIR PUMP, GAS-FORCED INFUSION, AND FLUIDICS

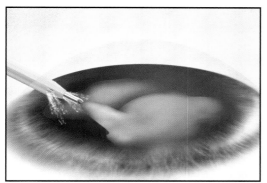

Figure 3-12. C-MICS. (Photo courtesy of Dr. Agarwal's Group of Eye Hospitals and Eye Research Centre, Chennai, India.)

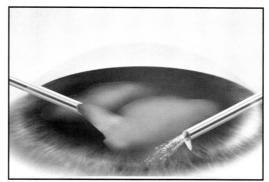

Figure 3-13. B-MICS. (Photo courtesy of Dr. Agarwal's Group of Eye Hospitals and Eye Research Centre, Chennai, India.)

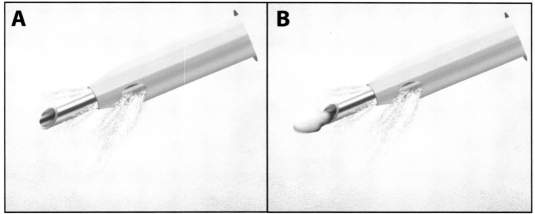

Figure 3-14. Fluidics in C-MICS. (A) Fluid flow. (B) Nuclear fragments pushed away. (Photo courtesy of Dr. Agarwal's Group of Eye Hospitals and Eye Research Centre, Chennai, India.)

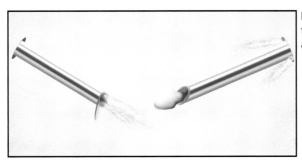

Figure 3-15. Fluidics in B-MICS. (Photo courtesy of Dr. Agarwal's Group of Eye Hospitals and Eye Research Centre, Chennai, India.)

With B-MICS, it is also possible to direct the irrigating chopper port toward the posterior capsule, allowing the flow of infusion solution to press down on that capsule and reducing the risk of posterior capsule rupture. By pointing the phaco tip downward while emulsifying and aspirating the nucleus, it is thus possible to safely perform intracapsular phaco.

B-MICS allows the positional relationship between infusion and aspiration to be changed freely. The infusion port and the aspiration port can be moved independently upward or downward within the anterior capsule. This makes it possible to vary the flow of infusion solution considerably within the eye. The infusion flow can assist a variety of phacoemulsification procedures and can also be advantageous in cases that are particularly difficult and complicated.

DISCUSSION

Surge is defined as the volume of the fluid forced out of the eye into the aspiration line at the instant of occlusion break. When the phacoemulsification handpiece tip is occluded, flow is interrupted and vacuum builds up to its preset values. Additionally, the aspiration tubing may collapse in the presence of high vacuum levels. Emulsification of the occluding fragment clears the block and the fluid rushes into the aspiration line to neutralize the pressure difference created between the positive pressure in the anterior chamber and the negative pressure in the aspiration tubing. In addition, if the aspiration line tubing is not reinforced to prevent collapse (tubing compliance), the tubing, constricted during occlusion, expands on occlusion break. These factors cause a rush of fluid from the anterior chamber into the phaco probe. If surge is present, the fluid in the anterior chamber has not been replaced rapidly enough to prevent shallowing of the anterior chamber.

The maintenance of intraocular pressure (steady-state IOP)[7] during the entire procedure depends on the equilibrium between the fluid inflow and outflow. The steady-state pressure level is the mean pressure equilibrium between inflow and outflow volumes. In most phacoemulsification machines, fluid inflow is provided by gravitational flow of the fluid from the BSS bottle through the tubing to the anterior chamber. This is determined by the bottle height relative to the patient's eye, the diameter of the tubing, and, most importantly, the outflow of fluid from the eye through the aspiration tube and leakage from the wounds.[7]

The inflow volume can be increased by either increasing the bottle height or enlarging the diameter of the inflow tube. The intraocular pressure increases by 10 mm Hg for every 15-cm increase in bottle height above the eye.[10]

High steady-state IOPs increase phaco safety by raising the mean IOP level up and away from zero; that is, by delaying surge-related anterior chamber collapse.[7]

An air pump increases the amount of fluid inflow, thus making the steady-state IOP high. This deepens the anterior chamber, increasing the surgical space available for maneuvering, and thus prevents complications like posterior capsular tears and corneal endothelial damage. The phenomenon of surge is neutralized by rapid inflow of fluid at the time of occlusion break. The recovery to steady-state IOP is so prompt that no surge occurs and this enables the surgeon to remain in foot position 3 through the occlusion break. High-vacuum phacoemulsification/phakonit can be safely performed in hard brown cataracts using an air pump. Phacoemulsification or phakonit under topical or no anesthesia[1,11] can be safely done, neutralizing the positive vitreous pressure occurring due to squeezing of the eyelids.

SUMMARY

The air pump is a new device that helps to prevent surge. This prevents posterior capsular rupture, helps deepen the anterior chamber, and makes phacoemulsification and phakonit safe procedures even in hard cataracts.

REFERENCES

1. Agarwal S, Agarwal A, Apple DJ, et al. Phakonit and laser phakonit. In: Agarwal, ed. *Phacoemulsification, Laser Cataract Surgery and Foldable IOLs*. 2nd ed. New Delhi, India: Jaypee Brothers; 2000:204-216.
2. Agarwal A, Agarwal S, Agarwal A. Antichamber collapser. *J Cataract Refract Surg*. 2002;28(7):1085-1086.
3. Agarwal A, Agarwal S, Agarwal A Narang P, Narang S. Phakonit: phacoemulsification through a 0.9 mm incision. *J Cataract Refract Surg*. 2001;27(10):1548-1552.
4. Agarwal A, Trivedi RH, Jacob S, Agarwal A, Agarwal S. Microphakonit: 700 micron cataract surgery. *Clin Ophthalmol*. 2007;1(3):323-325.
5. Agarwal A, Kumar DA, Jacob S, Agarwal A. In vivo analysis of wound architecture in 700 micron microphakonit surgery. *J Cataract Refract Surg*. 2008;34(9):1554-1560.
6. Kelman CD. Phacoemulsification and aspiration: a new technique of cataract removal: a preliminary report. *Am J Ophthalmol*. 1967;64:23-25.
7. Wilbrandt HR. Comparative analysis of the fluidics of the AMO Prestige, Alcon Legacy, and Storz Premiere phacoemulsification systems. *J Cataract Refract Surg*. 1997;23(5):766-780.
8. Seibel SB. *Phacodynamics*. Thorofare, NJ: SLACK Incorporated; 1995.
9. Fishkind WJ. The phaco machine: how and why it acts and reacts? In: Agarwal S, Agarwal A, Apple DJ, et al, eds. *Four Volume Textbook of Ophthalmology*. New Delhi, India: Jaypee Brothers; 2000.
10. Seibel SB. The fluidics and physics of phaco. In: Agarwal S, Agarwal A, Apple DJ, et al, eds. *Phacoemulsification, Laser Cataract Surgery and Foldable IOLs*. 2nd ed. New Delhi, India: Jaypee Brothers; 2000:45-54.
11. Agarwal S, Agarwal A, Apple DJ, et al. No-anaesthesia cataract surgery with karate chop. In: Agarwal S, Agarwal A, Apple DJ, et al, eds. *Phacoemulsification, Laser Cataract Surgery and Foldable IOLs*. 2nd ed. New Delhi, India: Jaypee Brothers; 2000:217-226.

SECTION II
MACHINES AND INSTRUMENTATION

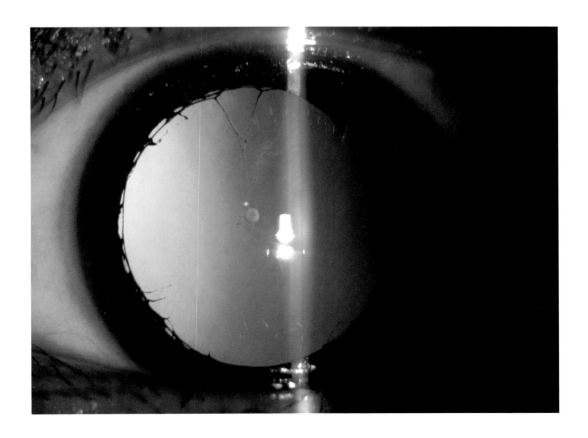

CHAPTER 4

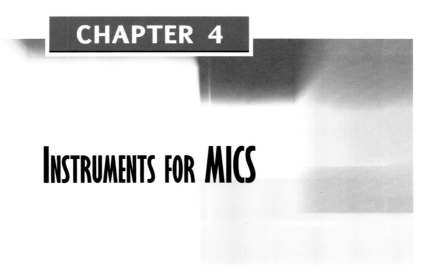

INSTRUMENTS FOR MICS

L. Felipe Vejarano, MD

Since the beginning of microincisional cataract surgery (MICS) in 1998 by Dr. Amar Agarwal (who started with a needle and an air pump), instrumentation has changed tremendously.[1-5]

INCISION

As in any kind of phacoemulsification technique (coaxial or bimanual MICS; C-MICS and B-MICS, respectively) the incision is one of the key points for the success of the procedure, particularly in microincision, because fluidics plays a very important role in the stability of the anterior chamber during surgery.[6-9] If the incision is too small, manipulation of the instruments produces corneal damage, impeding self-sealing of the incision. There is also difficulty in maneuvering the instrument into the eye. If the incision is too large, it can produce excessive leakage, causing instability of the anterior chamber and leading to collapse and endothelial damage. The incision tunnel length is also important and should be at least 1.5 mm so that there is no iris prolapse, especially when gas-forced infusion is on.

One should also know the diameter of the tip of the phaco needle to calculate the size of the incision and the diameter of the irrigation instrument (chopper most of the time) for the side port incision. The needle and the chopper are made of a metallic rigid circumference and the incision is a longitudinal elastic line. One calculates the circumference length of the instrument using the formula $2\pi r$, where r means radius of the instrument in mm. Each lip of the incision covers half of the instrument, so one has to divide the result by 2. Moreover, the cornea is an elastic tissue and one has to take into account the tissue compliance, which is calculated at approximately 20%. Thus, the final formula to decide upon the right size of the incision is:

$(2\pi r/2) - 20\%$; that is to say: $\pi \times r \times 0.80$.

As an example, if one is going to use a 1.067-mm outer diameter needle or irrigating chopper (19 gauge), the calculation for the main and side port incisions will be as follows:

$(\pi \times 0.533 \text{ mm}) = 1.674 \text{ mm} \times 0.80 = 1.33 \text{ mm}$

The sizes of the incision and the gauges of the phaco needles are shown in Table 4-1.

Table 4-1		
SIZE OF THE INCISION AND GAUGE OF THE INSTRUMENTS		
GAUGE	MILLIMETERS	INCISION (MM)
18	1.245	1.50
19	1.067	1.33
20	0.889	1.11
21	0.759	0.91
22	0.711	0.89

KNIVES

The author uses the nanotip for 700-µm cataract surgery (Figure 4-1) and Vejarano's irrigating chopper (MicroSurgical Technology, Redmond, WA; Figure 4-2), both 22 gauge, using a 1-mm diamond knife (Accutome, Malvern, PA; Figure 4-3) for the technique known as Vejarano's safe chop.[10-18] One can use a 1-mm steel lancet too (Alcon, Fort Worth, TX) or the 0.8-mm microphakonit knife (MicroSurgical Technology; Figure 4-4) designed by Amar Agarwal for 700-µm cataract surgery.

VISCOELASTICS

In this technique (microincision), one can use any kind of viscoelastic: cohesive, dispersive, or viscoadaptative. Because the incision size is small, the anterior chamber is well maintained. Thus, enough space is there during the rhexis.

CAPSULORRHEXIS

As in coaxial phaco, capsulorrhexis is the most important step in the whole surgery. An advantage of this technique is that you can switch your hands and use the micro-Utrata through the main or side port incision to facilitate success in this step. The micro-Utrata forceps has to be smaller than the incision size. A very good microrhexis forceps is made by MicroSurgical Technology—25-gauge microrhexis forceps (Figure 4-5). There are many other micro-Utrata forceps from other commercial manufacturers. The points to look for in a microrhexis forceps are:

* Direct action
* Curved arm
* Small tips even when the jaws are open or closed. This feature helps to avoid the lock at the internal lip of the incision with the joint between the cylinder of the forceps and its tips causing a focal Descemet's detachment.
* Sharp end tips to facilitate the tear of the anterior capsule, providing an easy grasp of the first flap of the rhexis.

If one develops a small rhexis, this can be enlarged using Microscissors (MicroSurgical Technology; Figure 4-6) 21 or 23 gauge. This helps to create and edge in the rhexis and then one can switch to the microrhexis forceps to complete the rhexis. The advantage of a microincision is the possibility of using any of the microinstruments through any of the incisions (Figure 4-7).

INSTRUMENTS FOR MICS

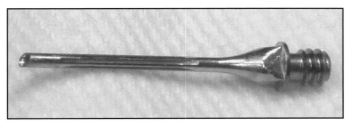

Figure 4-1. Agarwal's 700-μm phaco needle for microphakonit or microbiaxial surgery (MicroSurgical Technology). (Reprinted with permission from MicroSurgical Technology, Redmond, WA.)

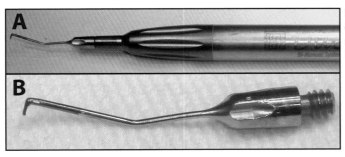

Figure 4-2. Vejarano irrigating chopper. (Reprinted with permission from MicroSurgical Technology, Redmond, WA.)

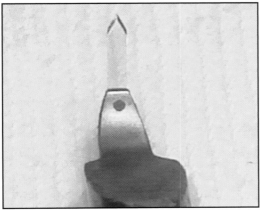

Figure 4-3. 1-mm diamond knife. (Photo courtesy of L. Felipe Vejarano.)

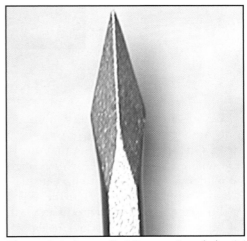

Figure 4-4. Agarwal's 0.8-mm microphakonit/microbiaxial knife. (Reprinted with permission from MicroSurgical Technology, Redmond, WA.)

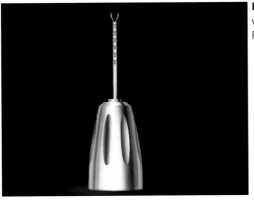

Figure 4-5. 25-gauge microrhexis forceps. (Reprinted with permission from MicroSurgical Technology, Redmond, WA.)

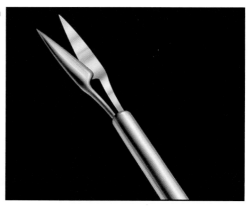

Figure 4-6. Microscissor. (Reprinted with permission from MicroSurgical Technology, Redmond, WA.)

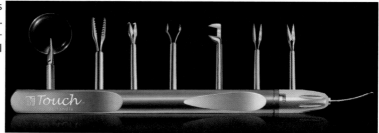

Figure 4-7. Microinstruments (MicroSurgical Technology). (Reprinted with permission from MicroSurgical Technology, Redmond, WA.)

Hydrodissection

Before one starts hydrodissection, one should remove some viscoelastic from the anterior chamber to avoid excess of pressure and rupture of the posterior capsule with a nucleus drop. One should remember that one is working in a small space, so the cannula has to be the smallest gauge possible with enough flow—for example, 26 or 27 gauge—but also easy to maneuver, so it is best to have a curved or angled cannula. A good cannula to use is the Chang cannula (Katena, Denville, NJ), 27 gauge (Figure 4-8). The author usually uses the technique of one-step hydrodissection, in which an anhydric dissection is made, followed by lifting of the anterior capsule with the cannula and separating it from the anterior cortex. Then, 2 or 3 mm from the rhexis edge toward the equator, a stream of balanced salt solution (BSS) is applied, always constant and at the same pressure. Once the wave below the nucleus is visible, fluid injection continues until a wave develops 180 degrees away from where you began. At this time, the BSS injection is stopped. At the opposite border of the rhexis, the nucleus is pushed back, making the fluid under the nucleus flow anteriorly and leave the bag. All of the adhesions between the cortex and capsule are removed and the nucleus can be rotated easily.

Phaco Needles

The standard 19-gauge phaco needle (Alcon) has an outer diameter of 1.12 mm and an inner diameter of 0.91 mm. The MicroFlow tip (Bausch & Lomb, Aliso Viejo, CA), designed by Barrett,[19] has an outer diameter of 1.07 mm (similar to a standard phaco needle) and, although it has an inner diameter of 0.9 mm at the end of the tip (again, similar to a standard phaco needle), it has a smaller shaft inner diameter (0.5 mm). The nanotip 22 gauge designed by Amar Agarwal (see Figures 2-1A and B; for B-MICS; MicroSurgical Technology) has an outer diameter of 0.7 mm and an inner diameter of 0.65 mm.

Figure 4-8. Chang's hydrodissection cannula. (Photo courtesy of L. Felipe Vejarano.)

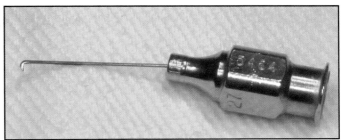

IRRIGATION CHOPPERS

There are 3 kinds of irrigation choppers, which differ on the stream of irrigation: frontal, inferior, and lateral in different gauges. MicroSurgical Technology has many irrigating choppers named after their designers (Figure 4-9). Each one has advantages and disadvantages:

* Frontal
  * Advantages
    * Good inflow
    * Good gauge
    * Good size of the side port incision
  * Disadvantages
    * Excessive turbulence
    * Rejects pieces from the phaco needle
    * Tissue trauma
    * Introduction technically difficult
* Inferior
  * Advantages
    * Best fluid circulation in the anterior chamber
  * Disadvantages
    * Lowest inflow related to gauge
    * Largest gauge to improve inflow
    * Large side port incision
    * Introduction technically difficult
* Lateral
  * Advantages
    * Enough inflow, 70% to 77%, compared to frontal
    * 75% to 85% inflow compared to inferior (largest gauge)
    * Good gauge
    * Good size of the side port incision
    * Minimal turbulence
    * Good fluid circulation in the anterior chamber
    * Stability of the anterior chamber
  * Disadvantages
    * Has insufficient inflow in very high vacuum

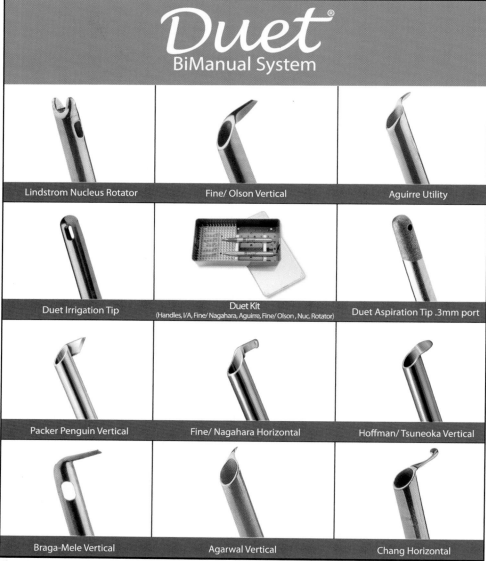

Figure 4-9. Irrigating choppers (Duet system, MicroSurgical Technology). (Reprinted with permission from MicroSurgical Technology, Redmond, WA.)

IRRIGATION/ASPIRATION

The most common in B-MICS are 20 gauge; in micro-B-MICS (microphakonit), the most common is the 22 gauge designed by Amar Agarwal (Figure 4-10). The aspiration handpiece has a polishing tip to help clean the posterior capsule and the epithelial cells from the anterior capsule (MicroSurgical Technology).

SUMMARY

Good instruments are crucial for surgery.

INSTRUMENTS FOR MICS

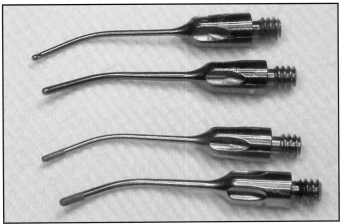

Figure 4-10. Agarwal's microphakonit 700-µm irrigating/aspirating cannula (MicroSurgical Technology). (Reprinted with permission from MicroSurgical Technology, Redmond, WA.)

REFERENCES

1. Tsuneoka H, Shiba T, Takahashi Y. Ultrasonic phacoemulsification using a 1.4 mm incision: clinical results. *J Cataract Refract Surg.* 2002;28(1):81-86.
2. Blumenthal M, Assia E, Chen V, Avni I. Using an anterior chamber maintainer to control intraocular pressure during phacoemulsification. *J Cataract Refract Surg.* 1994;20(1):93-96.
3. Agarwal A, Agarwal S, Agarwal A. Antichamber collapser. *J Cataract Refract Surg.* 2002;28(7):1085-1086.
4. Agarwal S, Chaudhry R, Chaudhry S. Bomba anticolapso de cámara. In: Boyd BF, Boyd S, eds. *Fako, Fakonit y Fako con Láser.* Panama: Highlights of Ophthalmology International; 2002.
5. Vejarano LF, Fine IH, Packer M, et al. MICS instrumentation growing in versatility, variety. *Ocul Surg News.* 2004;22(11):26-27.
6. Vejarano LF, Tello A. Fluidics in bimanual phaco. In: Agarwal A, ed. *Bimanual Phaco: Mastering the Phakonit/MICS Technique.* Thorofare, NJ: SLACK Incorporated; 2004:23-30.
7. Vejarano LF, Vejarano A, Tello A. Fluidics in phakonit. In: Garg A, ed. *Mastering the Art of Bimanual Microincision Phaco (Phaconit/MICS).* New Delhi, India: Jaypee Brothers; 2005:169-182.
8. Vejarano LF, Vejarano A, Tello A. Fluidics in phakonit and microphakonit. In: Garg A, ed. *Mastering the Phacodynamics (Tools, Technology and Innovations).* New Delhi, India: Jaypee Brothers; 2007:344-360.
9. Vejarano LF, Vejarano A, Tello A, Bovet J. Fluidics in biaxial lens surgery. In: Perez-Arteaga A, ed. *Step by Step Biaxial Lens Surgery.* New Delhi, India: Jaypee Brothers; 2008:95-135.
10. Vejarano LF, Tello A, Vejarano A, Vejarano M. The safer and most effective techniques in cataract surgery. *Highlights of Ophthalmology, International English Edition.* 2004;32(2):10-16.
11. Vejarano LF, Tello A, Vejarano A, Vejarano M. La técnica más segura y efectiva de Microincisión en cirugía de catarata. *Highlights of Ophthalmology, Edición para Hispanoamérica.* 2004;32(2):13-19.
12. Vejarano LF, Vejarano A, Vejarano M, Tello A. Faconit, una técnica de microincisión segura y efectiva en cirugía de cataratas. *Franja Ocular.* 2004;5(31):10-16.
13. Vejarano LF, Tello A. Vejarano's safe chop makes transition to chopping easier. *Ocul Surg News.* 2005;23(5):10-11.
14. Vejarano LF, Tello A. Vejarano's safe chop technique: a safer chopping. *Tech Ophthalmol.* 2005;3(3):109-115.
15. Vejarano LF, Vejarano A. Safe chopping in bimanual phaco. In: Agarwal A, ed. *Bimanual Phaco: Mastering the Phakonit/MICS Technique.* Thorofare, NJ: SLACK Incorporated; 2004:127-134.
16. Vejarano LF, Vejarano A, Tello A. Implantation techniques in microphaco: Vejarano's safe chop in phakonit. In: Garg A, ed. *Mastering the Art of Bimanual Microincision Phaco (Phaconit/MICS).* New Delhi, India: Jaypee Brothers; 2005:205-214.
17. Vejarano LF, Tello A, Vejarano A. Safe chop: a safer technique in phaco chop. In: Boyd S, Dodick J, eds. *New Outcomes in Cataract Surgery.* Ciudad de Panamá, Panamá: Highlights of Ophthalmology; 2005:71-76.
18. Vejarano LF, Tello A. Using safe horizontal chopping to prevent ruptures. In: Agarwal A, ed. *Phaco Nightmares.* Thorofare, NJ: SLACK Incorporated; 2006:53-64.
19. Barrett GD. Improved fluid dynamics during phacoemulsification with a new (MicroFlow) needle design. Paper presented at: ASCRS Symposium on Cataract, IOL and Refractive Surgery: Seattle, WA; June 1-5, 1996.

MICS Using Torsional Phacoemulsification and the Alcon INFINITI Vision System

Khiun F. Tjia, MD

Torsional ultrasound has indeed contributed significantly to microincisional cataract surgery (MICS).[1-3]

History and Development

As conventional phacoemulsification instrumentation has evolved, both ultrasonic and fluidic technologies have become more sophisticated. During this process, there have been ongoing efforts to develop other forms of tip motion to aid or replace the longitudinal motion of the traditional phacoemulsification ultrasound handpiece.

Alcon (Fort Worth, TX) introduced NeoSoniX in 2001 on the Legacy series console, which provides a 5-degree rotational movement of the phaco tip with an oscillatory frequency of 100 Hz, in addition to the traditional longitudinal ultrasound with a frequency of 40 000 Hz. It became popular because this sonic motion could be used to constantly reposition lens material on the phaco tip, which is especially beneficial for more efficient phacoemulsification of dense cataracts. However, the low-frequency oscillatory movement by itself was not the primary force that resulted in nucleus emulsification, and this made it mandatory for the modality to be used in conjunction with traditional, longitudinal ultrasound. Disassembly of the lens was still accomplished by the longitudinal tip movement, and the oscillatory motion functioned to constantly reposition dense fragments on the tip. The latter motion dramatically reduced the potential for "skewering" into the nucleus and thereby reduced the need for manipulations with a second instrument to release the impaled nucleus. The combination of an electric motor and a piezoelectric component resulted in a larger and heavier handpiece.

Five years of research and design engineering followed, culminating in 2006 with the introduction of the OZil torsional handpiece (Alcon), which enabled torsional phacoemulsification. An entirely new ultrasonic movement and concept was incorporated into this handpiece, electronic hardware, and software technology.

CHAPTER 5
CONVENTIONAL VERSUS TORSIONAL ULTRASOUND

Conventional longitudinal phacoemulsification relies on a titanium rod referred to as a *horn* that vibrates in resonance with the piezoelectric elements contained within the handpiece (Figure 5-1). The design requires that vibrations inside the handpiece be minimized and increase dramatically at the phaco tip, which is securely attached to the horn. Longitudinal vibrations occur along the handpiece. In contrast, the torsional modality causes the horn to twist so that the tip oscillates or rotates around its axis, similar to the motion of the NeoSoniX system, but at an ultrasonic frequency that induces lens fragmentation.

The provision of differing resonant frequencies for the longitudinal and torsional motion was critical; this permitted independent and separate ultrasound control having a signal at one frequency to induce only longitudinal motion and another signal at a different frequency to induce only torsional movement. The resonant frequencies must differ sufficiently so that cross talk—that is, unintended excitation of one mode when the other is activated—is prevented. The current torsional frequency of the OZil torsional handpiece of 32 kHz is separated from the longitudinal frequency of 43 kHz by 11 kHz, which is approximately 10 times greater than the width of each of the resonances.

As the horn and the phaco tip oscillate around their axes, the extremely high stress induced in the tip also causes it to twist. Figure 5-1 is therefore a simplistic geometric approximation of the actual tip motion.

With longitudinal phacoemulsification, lens fracturing is achieved by mechanical impact of the tip against the lens, known as the *jackhammer effect*.[4] The impact causes compression stress and eventual emulsification of lens material. However, the process inevitably causes repulsion, which is especially true with dense lens material because the tip stroke (power) must be lengthened to penetrate such lenses. Cutting/fracturing efficiency is reduced by this repellent effect, and an even greater power level may be required. This further increases lens repulsion (chatter) and leads to further loss of cutting efficiency.

Software programs have therefore been developed to modulate ultrasound delivery to reduce repulsion and permit some dissipation of thermal energy. This typically consists of intermittently delivering pulsed ultrasound, and although this can be helpful in increasing cutting efficacy and reducing both heat and repulsion, it slows the lens removal process.

With torsional ultrasound, cutting is generated by shearing at the surface of the lens. The tip movement causes no repulsion, and the creation of excessive frictional thermal energy within the incision is less of a concern. Interruption of energy is therefore of less importance, energy delivery can be constant, and this increases the efficiency of lens removal. In addition, unlike traditional phacoemulsification, during which the forward stroke can fracture the lens and the backward stroke produces no useful effect (yet contributes equally to heat generation at the incision), torsional phacoemulsification provides cutting when the tip moves to the left or right, effectively doubling its efficiency.

In a study comparing emulsification of dense nuclei by longitudinal or torsional ultrasound by measuring the fluid volume required to remove the nucleus, longitudinal phacoemulsification was found to require 50% more balanced salt solution than torsional phacoemulsification.[5]

The oscillatory movement of the torsional tip is highly effective in shaving lens material. However, when a flared tip design is used, the mechanism does not cause aspirated material to be jackhammered into and through the tip as it is with traditional phacoemulsification. Therefore, it is important for the material to be broken up into relatively small pieces that can pass through the inner lumen of the tip without obstructing it. If torsional

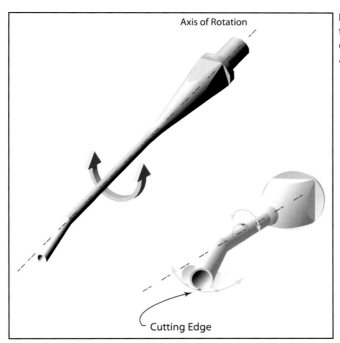

Figure 5-1. Comparison of cutting effectiveness. (Photo courtesy of Dr. Vaishali Vasavada, Memnagar, Ahmedabad, India.)

vibration is interrupted and/or larger fragments of dense lens material enter the lumen, tip obstruction may result. In such circumstances, elimination of the obstruction can be readily achieved by the addition of brief periods of longitudinal tip vibration. Alternatively, use of torsional ultrasound continuously above a certain threshold dramatically reduces the likelihood of tip clogging.

When an angulated tip is used, displacement at its distal portion is significantly larger than it would be with a straight tip. This is an important principle because the angulated design therefore reduces the amount of thermal energy dissipated at the incision site relative to the amount of energy delivered at the tip. Because ultrasonic energy released into the anterior chamber is distributed over a relatively large volume of surrounding fluid, insignificant temperature elevation within the anterior chamber occurs during phacoemulsification. Frictional heat created at the incision site, however, has a relatively small amount of fluid in its vicinity to dissipate thermal energy. Heat generated by friction between the vibrating tip and the surrounding sleeve is therefore capable of rapidly causing thermal injury to the surrounding tissues.

The velocity of the phaco tip is directly related to its ability to generate thermal energy. Tip velocity is determined by both the length of each stroke and the frequency of tip vibration. Traditional longitudinal ultrasound is delivered at 40 kHz, with a maximum of 90 μm of stoke length. The lower frequency of torsional ultrasound, 32 kHz, results in a reduction of temperature elevation at the incision by approximately 20%. In addition, the geometry of an angulated tip decreases the displacement of the tip at the incision relative to the displacement of its cutting edge. Depending on the phaco tip design, the latter results in an additional reduction in temperature increase at the incision.[6,7]

However, torsional motion is not only a more efficient modality from a thermal standpoint but also a more efficient one because the oscillatory tip motion causes little if any repulsion of lens material, resulting in more efficient emulsification.[8]

Anterior Chamber Stability With Torsional Ultrasound

Because of the shearing action of the torsional tip, sustained and uninterrupted lens removal occurs. This motion creates constant mini-occlusion breaks, resulting in lower effective vacuum levels throughout the emulsification of the lens. This leads to a more stable anterior chamber and lower pressure variance.[9,10] The use of relatively high flow and vacuum limits are not necessary with torsional ultrasound. Elevation of fluidic parameters is often required even with micropulsed longitudinal ultrasound to provide greater flow to the tip, attract chattering particles, and accelerate vacuum buildup during tip occlusion (the use of higher vacuum increases the holding force of the tip on the lens, thereby reducing repulsion).

Although higher flow and vacuum settings can accelerate lens removal with torsional ultrasound, elevation of these parameters to relatively high levels is not as important to the removal process. Christer Johansson, MD demonstrated that reduction of vacuum limit from 500 to 350 mm Hg did not cause an appreciable change in either the cumulative dissipated energy value or the removal time.[11]

Anterior chamber stability has been further improved with the introduction of the Intrepid Fluidic Management System (FMS; Alcon), a significantly lower compliance tubing system compared with the original FMS system. At moderate vacuum levels (ie, 300 to 350 mm Hg) currently widely used with the INFINITI Vision System (Alcon), the surge flow volume on occlusion break is extremely low with the Intrepid FMS compared with the regular FMS.

Effect of Tip Design

Standard surgical techniques and conventional phacoemulsification tips can be used with torsional ultrasound. However, angulated tips (Kelman tips; Alcon) amplify tip movement and cutting efficacy. This is particularly true of the Mini-Flared MicroTip (Alcon). A comparison of the performance of several tip designs is shown in Table 5-1.

STRAIGHT VERSUS BENT TIP

As explained above, an angled tip provides both greater displacement of the cutting edge and thermal benefits. It also facilitates tip depression without requiring handpiece elevation, and the tip can be repositioned within the anterior chamber by rotating the handpiece around the axis of the shaft; doing so may reduce the amount of stress placed on the incision during phacoemulsification. Angled tips of 12 to 20 degrees are available. Although the former produces 30% less amplification of movement at the distal tip, this design is suitable for surgeons who prefer a relatively straight tip.

A microcoaxial technique using an incision that results in minimized surgically induced astigmatism can be used in combination with a phaco tip and sleeve that provide an optimum fit for the incision size. For example, a Mini-Flared tip can be used with the Ultra Sleeve (Alcon) (2.2-mm incision).

Bent tips with the larger angulation of 20 degrees have potentially larger displacement at the cutting edge. In the most simplified geometric consideration, the larger the bend angle is, the greater oscillatory displacement is for a given rotational angle. The greater the tip movement is, the more resistance it encounters as it moves through fluid. As a result, the tip's shaft twists, which diminishes the amount of displacement at the cutting edge. Greater mass at the tip's edge further increases shaft twisting and reduces movement at the edge. Reducing the tip diameter or the tip wall thickness makes the twisting more pronounced.

Table 5-1
PHACO TIP DESIGNS AND TORSIONAL PERFORMANCE

STROKE	TAPERED KELMAN	MINI-FLARED OZIL 12	MINI-FLARED REVERSE OZIL 12	1.1 FLARED REVERSE OZIL 12	MINI-FLARED KELMAN
At cutting edge	90 μm*	100 μm*	100 μm*	130 μm*	130 μm*
At incision†	40 μm*	40 μm*	30 μm*	50 μm*	40 μm*
Incision/cutting edge ratio (%)	40‡	40‡	30‡	40‡	30‡

*Rounded to the nearest 10 μm.
†Stroke measured at approximately 5.6 mm from the cutting edge.
‡Rounded to the nearest 10%.

Thus, one can see that optimizing torsional tip performance is a complicated task that requires careful consideration of many variables, all of which also affect fluidics performance of the tip.

Reducing the bend angle from 20 to 12 degrees reduces the displacement at the cutting edge, but it still provides very good torsional performance in the Mini-Flared configuration as shown in Table 5-2. At the same time, the reduced angle may provide a greater ergonomic advantage that is acceptable to many surgeons.

TIP BEVEL

All tips are available with either 30- or 45-degree bevels; however, the 45-degree variety excels with torsional. Its sharper tip provides enhanced cutting, especially during nucleus sculpting. The larger opening of a 45-degree tip also removes a softer nucleus more rapidly because greater holding force on the nucleus occurs during tip occlusion.

The greater bevel may also induce more repositioning of dense lens material on the tip. This prevents "coring" of the nucleus and, therefore, the need to frequently reposition lens material with a second instrument. The increased cutting of lens material may reduce the possibility of tip obstruction.[12]

Although it is easier to impale the nucleus with a 30-degree tip, this maneuver can be facilitated with either a 30- or 45-degree tip by orienting the port in a horizontal fashion.

Additional phaco tip designs have been developed following ideas independently proposed by Takuyki Akahoshi, MD and Robert Osher, MD. These tips used a reverse 30-degree tip (Figure 5-2) with a reduced tip angulation of 12 degrees to provide enhanced occlusion during sculpting. The tip can be oriented horizontally during nuclear segment removal. The tip preferred by both surgeons is based on a 1.1-mm flared tip design, and many surgeons prefer smaller openings.

To accommodate this preference, an alternative tip was developed based on the Mini-Flared MicroTip but also featuring a reverse bevel of 30 degrees and a reduced bend angle of 12 degrees.

ULTRASONIC TIP AND SLEEVE DESIGN

Both infusion sleeve and phaco tip design are critically important to the performance of phacoemulsification equipment. These items have variable length, inner diameter, and outer diameter, and are designed to function best with certain types of tips. Console parameters—vacuum limit, flow rate, dynamic rise, and infusion bottle height—must be appropriate for the tip and sleeve used.

Table 5-2

PHACO TIP DESIGNS AND FLUIDICS PERFORMANCE

Tip	Vacuum*	Port Area	Holding Force	Microcoaxial
Mini-Flared MicroTip	High	Medium	High	High
MicroTip (0.9 mm)	Medium	Medium	Medium	Medium
Tapered MicroTip	Medium	Large	Medium	Medium
Mackool MicroTip	Medium	Medium	Medium	Medium
Standard (1.1 mm)	Low	Large	Medium	Low

*Relative level of vacuum that can be used, as determined by the infusion capacity and shaft internal diameter of the various tip/sleeve combinations.

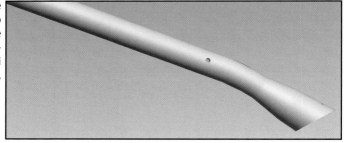

Figure 5-2. Phaco tip with a reverse 30-degree tip and a reduced tip angulation of 12 degrees to provide enhanced occlusion during sculpting. (Photo courtesy of Dr. Vaishali Vasavada, Memnagar, Ahmedabad, India.)

The INFINITI Vision System uses 2 categories of tips and sleeves, MicroTip (0.9 mm) and standard (1.1 mm), with several variations of each (Table 5-3):

* The infusion capacities and dimensions of the various 0.9-mm infusion sleeves when used in combination with a Mini-Flared tip are shown in Table 5-4.
* The high-infusion sleeve (HIS) provides the greatest infusion capacity, which is 38% greater than the capacity attainable with an Ultra Sleeve.
* The infusion capacity and dimensions of the 1.1-mm various infusion sleeve designs when used in combination with a 1.1-mm flared tip are shown in Table 5-5.
* The HIS again provides the greatest infusion capacity, which is approximately 58% greater than the capacity attainable with an Ultra Sleeve.

OZIL IP SOFTWARE

In September 2009, a new software upgrade was released. OZil IP software allows the user to momentarily supplement torsional amplitude with brief bursts of longitudinal ultrasound when a programmable vacuum threshold is exceeded. These short bursts of conventional ultrasound help to minimize occlusions and hence further improve fluidic stability. They also help to keep nuclear material at the ideal position of the phaco tip end, where the shaving action of torsional ultrasound occurs. The OZil IP feature can be enabled for each individual procedure step and for each cataract grade.

Table 5-3

INFINITI VISION SYSTEM TIPS AND SLEEVES COMBINATIONS*

	ULTRASOUND TIPS	COMPATIBLE INFUSION SLEEVES
MicroTip (0.9 mm)	Mini-Flared (purple)	Ultra (rose)
	MicroTip (purple)	Micro (dark purple)
	Tapered MicroTip (purple)	High infusion (light purple)
	MicroTip ABS (purple)	
Standard (1.1 mm)	Standard (blue)	Ultra (green)
	Standard ABS (distal blue)	Micro (green blue)
	Standard flared ABS (distal blue)	Standard (dark blue)
		High infusion (light purple)

*The MicroTip and Tapered MicroTip have a 0.1-mm larger shaft diameter than the Mini-Flared tip. Their infusion capacity is therefore reduced in comparison with the latter.

Table 5-4

0.9-MM INFUSION SLEEVES AND IRRIGATION FLOW PERFORMANCE

	0.9-MM INFUSION SLEEVES		
	*HIS**	*Micro*	*Ultra*
Free flow, mL/min†	84	70	61
Shaft OD, mm	2.2	2.0	1.8
Shaft ID, mm	1.8	1.6	1.4
Front OD, mm	1.2	1.2	1.2
Front ID, mm	1.0	1.0	1.0
Port ID, mm	1.2	1.0	1.0

*HIS indicates high infusion sleeve; ID, inner diameter; OD, outer diameter.
†Infusion bottle height 78 cm.

Table 5-5

1.1-MM INFUSION SLEEVES AND IRRIGATION FLOW PERFORMANCE

	1.1-MM INFUSION SLEEVES			
	*HIS**	*1.1 mm*	*Micro*	*Ultra*
Free flow, mL/min†	93	87	84	65
Shaft OD, mm	2.1	2.0	2.0	1.8
Shaft ID, mm	1.7	1.6	1.6	1.4
Front OD, mm	1.4	1.4	1.4	1.4
Front ID, mm	1.2	1.2	1.2	1.2
Port ID, mm	1.4	1.4	1.2	1.2

*HIS indicates high infusion sleeve; ID, inner diameter; OD, outer diameter.
†Infusion bottle height 78 cm.

CHAPTER 5

TORSIONAL ULTRASOUND AND MICROINCISIONAL CATARACT SURGERY

The advantages of torsional ultrasound apply to both bimanual MICS (B-MICS) and coaxial MICS (C-MICS). Since 2005, C-MICS has gained considerable interest from surgeons around the world. In 2006, I stated that the nonrepulsive cutting action of torsional ultrasound perfectly matched the lower fluidics requirements of microcoaxial phaco and that this would have a dramatic effect on the adoption of microcoaxial phaco in the field of cataract surgery.[13] The transition from regular coaxial to microcoaxial torsional phaco has indeed proven to be easy, and microcoaxial torsional phacoemulsification is currently widespread.[14]

The fluidics settings adaptation for microcoaxial torsional phaco needs to be addressed: a reduction of incision size implicates a reduced sleeve size and results in proportional decreased irrigation flow capacity. This requires an adjustment of aspiration flow, the reduction of which should directly correlate to the reduction in irrigation flow.

With torsional ultrasound, efficiency of emulsification is still extremely efficient at low aspiration flow rates. The virtual lack of repulsion is responsible for the fact that routine phaco through microincisions is possible at modest fluidics settings. Dissipated energy, fluid use, and procedure time are comparable between regular coaxial and 2.2-mm microcoaxial phaco surgery.[15]

My personal fluidics settings for 2.2-mm microcoaxial torsional phaco in quadrant removal with the use of a Mini-Flared Kelman tip and Ultra Sleeve are shown in Table 5-6.

C-MICS through a 1.8-mm incision with the INFINITI machine has also been shown to be effective.[16,17] In 2009, the smaller Nano Sleeve (Alcon), required for 1.8-mm surgery, had not yet been released to the market. The only adjustment to fluidics settings would be a 10% to 15% reduction of aspiration flow (21 to 25 mL/min instead of 25 to 30 mL/min) with the use of the same 45 degree-Mini-Flared Kelman tip and Nano Sleeve. Alternatively, one could choose to raise the irrigation bottle to compensate for the decreased infusion capacity.

COAXIAL MICS WITH TORSIONAL ULTRASOUND IN VERY DENSE CATARACT CASES

Cataract surgery has become safer and much more efficient with the advent of torsional phacoemulsification. However, this technology is even more valuable when applied to very dense nuclei and other complex surgical situations.

Phacoemulsification of a dense lens always presents a greater challenge to surgeons. Dense nucleus removal with the use of longitudinal ultrasound requires more substantial and higher velocity impact of the vibrating metallic tip (jackhammer effect) to emulsify and remove the dense lens material. High fluidics settings are also required to offset repulsion of longitudinal ultrasound. This results in increased turbulence and fluid use and a higher incidence of corneal decompensation.

However, the side-to-side shearing action of torsional ultrasound has proven to be more efficient and effective at emulsifying lens material.[18] Torsional ultrasound is still effective at moderate vacuum settings and very-low-flow aspiration flow settings.[19] A very low aspiration flow (eg, 15 mL/min; Figure 5-3) will not aspirate a dispersive viscoelastic substance that protects the corneal endothelium. The combination of a dispersive viscoelastic and very-low-flow torsional phacoemulsification is my preferred strategy for very dense cataract surgery.[20]

Table 5-6	
SETTINGS FOR INFINITI MACHINE FOR ROUTINE CASES	
PERSONAL INFINITI PARAMETERS: ROUTINE CATARACT CASES	QUADRANT REMOVAL, 2.2-MM INCISION, MINI-FLARED TIP, INTREPID FMS*, ULTRA SLEEVE
Infusion bottle height	75-90 cm
Aspiration flow rate	25 mL/min fixed
Vacuum limit	300 mm Hg fixed
OZil amplitude	35% minimum-80% maximum linear

*FMS indicates fluid management system.

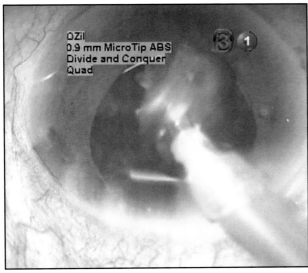

Figure 5-3. Aspiration flow of 15 mL/min in a very dense nucleus case.

INNOVATIVE PRECHOPPING DEVICE

Dividing a very dense nucleus is the most challenging part of the procedure. Luis Escaf, MD from Colombia developed an innovative ultrasonic-driven blade called the Ultrachopper (Alcon) that allows the division of nuclei of all densities with amazing ease.[21] The Ultrachopper is an ultrasonic knife similar to a phaco needle but with a flattened and tilted end. When driven by an OZil torsional handpiece in full torsional ultrasound mode, it creates a perfect vertical cut of approximately 100 µm with great ease and control. It is not yet commercially available.

TORSIONAL ULTRASONIC TIP SELECTION FOR DENSE NUCLEI

For a very dense nucleus, a 45-degree beveled tip is most efficient because the 45-degree beveled tip has a larger shearing surface and removes larger amounts of nuclear material than smaller diameter tips do. Also, the 45-degree bevel occludes less and repositions lens material on the vibrating tip, which proves very useful with dense lenses.

In general, a tip with a substantially flared design is more prone to unintentional obstruction of the tip and internal aspiration channel or shaft. This can lead to full or partial occlusion of the tip where insufficient tip cooling and possible thermal injury can result. Low-amplitude torsional ultrasound has a higher risk of tip clogging. Therefore, a high minimum amplitude setting of around 60% is recommended. A mix or blending of torsional and longitudinal ultrasound is often used by some surgeons to prevent or eliminate obstruction of the tip by very dense nuclear material. Also, surgeons should divide or chop the nucleus in smaller free pieces to allow easier tumbling and more efficient emulsification.

A MicroTip, with its nonflared design, has no likelihood of any internal obstruction because of its constant internal diameter throughout the length of the internal shaft of the tip. I therefore prefer a MicroTip for very dense (brown or black) nuclei and a Mini-Flared tip for soft- to medium-density lenses (Table 5-7).

COAXIAL MICS WITH TORSIONAL PHACOEMULSIFICATION IN OTHER COMPLEX CASES

Challenging and complicated conditions encountered during phacoemulsification include zonular weakness or dehiscence, posterior capsule rupture, floppy iris syndrome, and corneal endothelial dystrophy. In all of these situations, ocular turbulence can have a negative effect on the outcome.

A high aspiration flow rate, often used with traditional longitudinal phaco to reduce lens chatter, attracts vitreous or a floppy iris to the phaco tip. In addition, high flow and turbulence in the anterior chamber will evacuate viscoelastic, which reduces the protection of the endothelium during the procedure. The direct impact of mobile, chattering nuclear fragments also causes substantial turbulence and results in endothelial cell loss.

A higher vacuum level, also used to enhance efficiency with longitudinal ultrasound, may cause significant postocclusion surge at the time of occlusion break. This results in increased anterior chamber instability and intraocular pressure (IOP) fluctuations that can destabilize and escalate the danger of a complicated case. In instances of capsular rupture and an unstable chamber, nuclear fragments may shift or fall into the posterior segment. In a complicated case with an eye with zonular weakness and chamber instability, zonular dehiscence may develop or increase. Nonetheless, a certain amount of vacuum and flow is required to bring material efficiently to the phaco tip so that the surgeon can remove the dense nuclear material.

With traditional technology, a reduction of fluidic parameters can greatly diminish the holding power of the tip. This decreases the efficiency of the jackhammer effect and increases lens chatter, which results in nuclear fragment dispersal with increased turbulence within the eye. The controlled oscillatory, side-to-side motion of torsional ultrasound does not induce any significant repellent force. Because of this, nuclear material remains at the tip when energy is activated even at relatively low-flow/vacuum levels. Turbulence in the anterior chamber is reduced because of near constant contact of the tip with the nucleus even with a vibrating ultrasonic phaco tip. Both side-to-side motions of the torsional tip emulsify lens material. The lack of repulsion and increased emulsification combine to increase cutting efficiency with very dense lenses and reduce the time required for the procedure. I have found that I can use an aspiration flow rate of 12 to 15 mL/min, an infusion bottle height of 40 to 50 cm, and a vacuum setting of 250 to 300 mm Hg, which provide remarkably efficient nucleus removal with torsional phacoemulsification.

Table 5-7

SETTINGS FOR INFINITI MACHINE FOR DENSE CATARACT CASES

Personal INFINITI Parameters: Very Dense Cataracts	Quadrant Removal, 2.2-mm Incision, MicroTip, Intrepid FMS*, Ultra Sleeve
Infusion bottle height	75-90 cm
Aspiration flow rate	15 mL/min fixed
Vacuum limit	300 mm Hg fixed
OZil amplitude	50% minimum-100% maximum linear

*FMS indicates fluid management system.

Less turbulence and procedural time allow protective viscoelastic substances to be better retained, and the added retention results in increased protection of the corneal endothelium. Also, when zonular laxity, posterior capsule rupture, or floppy iris is encountered during a procedure, the greatly reduced turbulence and chamber stability of the lower fluidic settings decrease the likelihood of vitreous or iris attraction to the tip. A dispersive viscoelastic that has been injected to contain vitreous, position the iris, or retain the location of a nuclear fragment is not easily aspirated. A safe working distance can therefore be maintained between the phaco tip and the vitreous or iris.

ZONULAR WEAKNESS OR DEHISCENCE

In the presence of zonular laxity or deficiency, conservation of the structural integrity of the remaining fibers is important. Therefore, all aspects of the procedure should avoid stress to this delicate structure. The use of capsule retractors, hydrodissection and viscodissection, and nucleus rotation and disassembly must be performed with the utmost caution.

Intraocular pressure is greatest when the phaco tip is fully occluded, and it may drop precipitously with an occlusion break. Such rapid pressure changes can stress the zonule and can be minimized by lowering the infusion bottle and/or reducing the aspiration flow rate and maximum vacuum level. The lowered bottle reduces infusion capacity, which requires adjustment of fluidic settings. The aspiration flow rate can be reduced to 12 to 15 mL/min, and the vacuum limit should also be reduced to 250 mm Hg or below to maintain a low but stable IOP. Torsional phaco can be of great benefit because of the efficiency of emulsification at lower fluidic parameters, which allows minimal IOP fluctuations and fluidic turbulence.

INTRAOPERATIVE FLOPPY IRIS SYNDROME

Intraoperative floppy iris syndrome (discovered by David Chang) is characterized by a flaccid iris that billows and moves in response to fluid flow and movement. The iris has an increased tendency to migrate toward and prolapse through surgical incisions. This situation is also characterized by progressive intraoperative miosis, causing surgeons to have limited working space for phacoemulsification. Measures to stabilize and control the iris include preoperative topical atropine, intracameral phenylephrine, iris retractors, and viscoelastic injection. A nonturbulent, low-flow strategy, similar to that used in eyes with zonular weakness, can be valuable.[22] The lower fluidic parameters avoid iris attraction to the phaco tip, and a dispersive viscoelastic placed near the iris will not be readily evacuated.

The virtual absence of repulsion and attractability of lens tissue with torsional phacoemulsification reduces the need to pursue nuclear fragments even at these low fluidic parameters, and the phaco tip can be kept in the center of the pupil, above or below the iris plane. Phacoemulsification can be performed in a precise, controlled, and efficient fashion with a reduced tendency for the iris to billow or prolapse out of incisions.

POSTERIOR CAPSULE TEAR

If a posterior capsule tear occurs during nucleus removal, the handpiece should be left in the eye (foot pedal position zero) and a dispersive viscoelastic (ie, Viscoat, Alcon) should be injected behind the remaining lens segments. The dispersive viscoelastic seals and occludes/plugs the posterior capsule opening, which results in greater stabilization of the position of the lens material left to be emulsified. The remaining nucleus is then elevated to or above the iris plane, and the phaco tip is positioned beneath lens fragments. Then, careful emulsification with very low fluidics settings is used to remove the remaining lens material in a controlled manner without aspirating the underlying viscoelastic. Injection of additional viscoelastic permits each segment to be positioned appropriately and then removed without the creation of significant turbulence or viscoelastic aspiration, leaving the protective seal or plug in the ruptured area of the capsule (Table 5-8).

ACRYSOF SINGLE-PIECE INTRAOCULAR LENS INJECTION THROUGH 2.2-MM INCISIONS AND SMALLER

Cataract surgery has evolved since the development of ultrasonic emulsification in 1967. The introduction of foldable intraocular lenses (IOLs) in the early 1990s greatly impacted the reduction of incision sizes. The ongoing process to improve surgical outcomes and minimize complications is complemented by a further reduction in incision size. Wound-assisted IOL injection techniques were used by several surgeons in the mid-1990s. I personally started to use this technique in 1994 to slow down the unfolding of the trailing haptic of a silicone plate haptic IOL. When AcrySof Single-Piece IOLs (Alcon) became available, I began to use the wound-assisted injection technique (Figure 5-4) again to decrease incision size.[23] Takayuki Akahoshi, MD and I reported on sub-2.0-mm AcrySof IOL injection through Monarch C cartridges (Alcon; Figure 5-5) in 2005.[24] Dr. Akahoshi has described his countertraction technique for a 1.8-mm IOL injection.[25] In September 2007, the smaller D cartridge was introduced, which greatly facilitates 2.2-mm wound-assisted IOL injection.[26] With the D cartridge, wound stretch is limited and wound integrity is well preserved after IOL injection, resulting in watertight incisions. The aspheric AcrySof IQ has a 9% central thickness reduction compared with the nonaspheric lens. This makes the AcrySof IQ particularly well suited for MICS.

Some surgeons inject AcrySof IOLs through 1.8-mm incisions, but the majority of surgeons still operate through 2.2-mm or larger incisions. However, as technology evolves, we can surely expect the development of innovative IOL injection systems for smaller incisions in the future.

Table 5-8	
SETTINGS FOR INFINITI MACHINE FOR COMPLEX CATARACT CASES	
PERSONAL INFINITI PARAMETERS: COMPLEX CATARACT CASES	QUADRANT REMOVAL, 2.2-MM INCISION, MINI-FLARED TIP, INTREPID FMS*, ULTRA SLEEVE
Infusion bottle height	40-50 cm
Aspiration flow rate	12 mL/min linear
Vacuum limit	250-300 mm Hg fixed
OZil amplitude	35% minimum-80% maximum linear

*FMS indicates fluid management system.

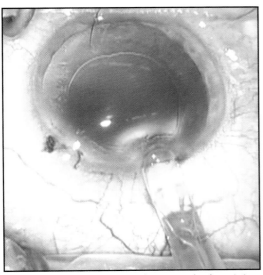

Figure 5-4. Wound-assisted intraocular lens injection, 2.2 mm with C cartridge.

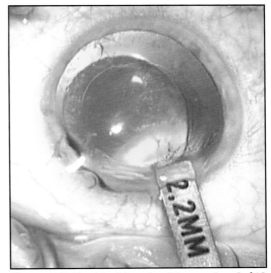

Figure 5-5. Final incision size 2.1 mm, AcrySof IQ intraocular lens with C cartridge.

SUMMARY

Torsional phacoemulsification represents a major advance in cataract removal technology. Numerous theoretical advantages have been confirmed by both laboratory investigations and clinical studies.

* The oscillatory direction of tip motion virtually eliminates repulsion of lens material.
* Frictional heat production between the phaco tip and sleeve at the incision is reduced.
* The handpiece is smaller and lighter than its predecessor, the NeoSoniX handpiece, which also offered oscillatory motion.
* The torsional handpiece can also be used to perform conventional phacoemulsification and can alternately deliver torsional and longitudinal motion.

* Torsional technology does not require alteration of surgical technique. Therefore, there is no significant learning curve.
* Transitioning to microcoaxial phacoemulsification (2.2 mm to 1.8 mm) requires an adjustment of fluidics settings. Because of the absence of repulsion, emulsification remains efficient.
* A low fluidics strategy with torsional ultrasound phacoemulsification is beneficial for very dense nuclei and other challenging cases.
* Wound-assisted AcrySof IOL injection through 2.2-mm incisions with the D cartridge is easy and preserves good wound integrity.
* Sub-2.0-mm AcrySof IOL injection is feasible but not yet common with current injection systems.

References

1. Tjia K. Torsional lens removal technology. Paper presented at: XXIII Congress of the ESCRS; September 13, 2005; Lisbon, Portugal.
2. Tjia K. Total cataract removal procedure through a 2.0-2.2 mm incision using new torsional lens removal technology and new smaller sleeves. Paper presented at: XXIII Congress of the ESCRS; September 13, 2005; Lisbon, Portugal.
3. Tjia K. Trends in phacoemulsification. *Ophthalmol Times Eur.* 2005;1:32-34.
4. Zacharias J. Role of cavitation in the phacoemulsification process. *J Cataract Refract Surg.* 2008;34(5):846-852.
5. Tjia K. Efficiency of torsional versus longitudinal ultrasound. *Cataract Refract Surg Today Eur.* 2008;3(4):33-34.
6. Hans Y, Miller K. Thermal imaging comparison of longitudinal versus torsional phacoemulsification in INFINITI. Paper presented at: ASCRS Symposium on Cataract, IOL and Refractive Surgery; April 3-8, 2009; San Francisco, CA.
7. Jun B, Berdahl JP, Kim T. Thermal study of longitudinal and torsional ultrasound phacoemulsification: tracking the temperature of corneal surface, incision and handpiece. Paper presented at: ASCRS Symposium on Cataract, IOL and Refractive Surgery; April 3-8, 2009; San Francisco, CA.
8. Davison JA. Cumulative tip travel and implied followability of longitudinal and torsional phacoemulsification. *J Cataract Refract Surg.* 2008;34(6):986-990.
9. Vasavada VA, Vasavada AR, Raj SM, Pandita D. Evaluation of enhanced fluidic pressure fluctuations during phacoemulsification using torsional ultrasound. Paper presented at: ASCRS Symposium on Cataract, IOL and Refractive Surgery; April 3-8, 2009; San Francisco, CA.
10. Vasavada AR, Pandita D, Raj SM. Comparing dynamic IOP measurements during phacoemulsification using traditional ultrasound versus torsional. Paper presented at: ASCRS Symposium on Cataract, IOL and Refractive Surgery; April 4-9, 2008; Chicago, IL.
11. Johansson C. Optimizing vacuum settings in torsional ultrasound phacoemulsification. *Cataract Refract Surg Today Eur.* 2008;3(4):24-27.
12. Allen D. Comparison of efficiency of 30° and 45° Mini-Flared Kelman tips during torsional phacoemulsification. Paper presented at: XXV Congress of the ESCRS; September 8, 2007; Stockholm, Sweden.
13. Tjia K. Microcoaxial phacoemulsification: a new standard in cataract surgery? *Cataract Refract Surg Today Eur.* 2006;1(2):18-20.
14. Tjia K. Routine use of microcoaxial torsional phaco. *Cataract Refract Surg Today Eur.* 2007;2(1):14-16.
15. Tjia K. Fluid use and ultrasound energy comparison between coaxial and micro-coaxial torsional ultrasound. Poster session presented at: XXVI Congress of the ESCRS; September 13-17, 2008; Berlin, Germany.
16. Packard R. Microcoaxial phaco with 1.8 mm incisions using 2 phaco machines and IOL systems. Paper presented at: XXVI Congress of the ESCRS; September 14, 2008; Berlin, Germany.
17. Tjia K. Is there an optimal incision size for routine cataract surgery? *Cataract Refract Surg Today Eur.* 2009;4(10):58-61.
18. Liu Y, Zeng M, Liu X, et al. Torsional mode versus conventional ultrasound mode phacoemulsification: randomized comparative clinical study. *J Cataract Refract Surg.* 2007;33(2):287-292.

19. Tjia K. A low fluidics parameters strategy. *Cataract Refract Surg Today Eur.* 2007;2(2):52-53.
20. Tjia K. Super-dense cataract surgery: low fluidics strategy for best patient outcomes. Paper presented at: ASCRS Symposium on Cataract, IOL and Refractive Surgery; April 5, 2009; San Francisco, CA.
21. Escaf L. A new way to divide the nucleus. *Cataract Refract Surg Today Eur.* 2007;2(2):32-36.
22. Tjia K. Unexpected IFIS cases: what should you do? *Cataract Refract Surg Today Eur.* 2009;4(3):54-55.
23. Tjia K. Small incision possible with single-piece lens injector system. *Ophthalmol Times.* 2003;28(6):47.
24. McGrath D. Innovations open door to sub 2.0 mm microcoaxial phaco. *EuroTimes.* 2005;9:7.
25. Akahoshi T. The counteraction technique: implanting a 6-mm Acrysof lens through a sub–2-mm incision. *Cataract Refract Surg Today Eur.* 2006;1(3):37-39.
26. Tjia K. Advances in microcoaxial phaco. *Cataract Refract Surg Today Eur.* 2007;2(7):21-22.

CHAPTER 6

1.8-mm Coaxial MICS With the Stellaris Platform

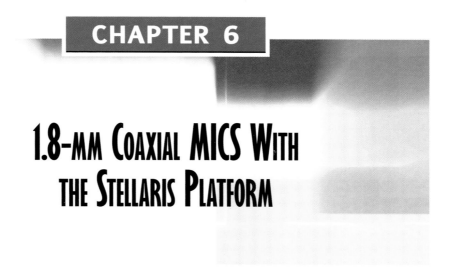

Terence M. Devine, MD

As phaco techniques have evolved from 3.5-mm incisions to below 2 mm,[1,2] a number of technologic challenges have been addressed. Some of these include fluidics control, chamber stability, optimizing ultrasonic power, and minimizing thermal risk of corneal burn. 1.8-mm coaxial microincisional cataract surgery (C-MICS) is a good technique to adopt.

Advantages of Coaxial Microincisional Surgery

Perhaps the greatest advantage of 1.8-mm C-MICS is that surgeons can achieve the benefits of sub-2-mm surgery with little or no learning curve. It is compatible with any technique and surgeons' familiar fluidics settings. It offers improved visibility and maneuverability, which benefits any case but is particularly helpful with small pupils, intraoperative floppy iris syndrome (IFIS), pseudoexfoliation, or situations with disrupted zonules or capsule. In contrast to bimanual MICS (B-MICS), C-MICS maintains the infusion sleeve to reduce leakage, improve chamber stability, and protect the cornea from friction and stress to improve the water-tight seal. The nondominant hand is not "pinned" inside the eye to maintain infusion and smaller, more ergonomic side-port instruments can be used. For these and other reasons, many surgeons have now adopted 1.8-mm C-MICS even if they plan to enlarge the incision for intraocular lens (IOL) insertion.

Fluidics Control

In terms of fluidics, the principle for safety is simple: inflow must always replace any outflow through the needle and any leakage through the incisions. The difficulty from an engineering perspective lies in the fact that the anterior chamber only contains approximately 0.3 mL or 6 drops of fluid. This means that if outflow exceeds inflow by 6 drops, the anterior chamber will collapse with potential damage to endothelium, capsule, and other intraocular tissues. This inflow/outflow balance must be maintained at all times but becomes most critical in the situation of postocclusion surge.

CHAPTER 6

Postocclusion surge occurs when an occluded phaco needle suddenly aspirates a piece of nucleus. The amount of fluid aspirated at that moment is related to several things:

* The internal diameter of the needle and aspiration tubing, which determine the resistance to outflow
* The tubing compliance or "stiffness." During occlusion, soft aspiration tubing will compress as vacuum rises and then rebound when the occlusion breaks, adding to the volume of fluid drawn from the anterior chamber
* The "pressure differential" when the needle is occluded. The pressure differential is the difference between the positive intraocular pressure (IOP) related to bottle height and the negative pressure inside the needle determined by vacuum level generated by the pump

The volume of aspirated surge fluid must be immediately replaced by infusion or the chamber will collapse. This fluidics challenge becomes amplified for sub-2-mm phaco because the smaller diameter infusion instruments for B-MICS, or the smaller infusion sleeves for C-MICS, will deliver less fluid per second for any given bottle height.

To overcome this limitation, one alternative is to use higher bottles to increase the potential infusion volume per second. Some surgeons have recommended using bottles as high as 150 cm. The problem with this approach is that IOP is directly proportional to bottle height and inversely proportional to outflow. Therefore, whenever aspiration is stopped either by tip occlusion or the surgeon returning to foot pedal position 1, the IOP is solely determined by the bottle height. Balanced salt solution (BSS) produces approximately 0.73 mm Hg pressure per cm of bottle height. Therefore, with no outflow, a 150-cm bottle height produces 110 mm Hg intraocular pressure.

The magnitude of IOP is only part of the concern. As aspiration is restored, the IOP will drop proportional to the outflow rate. During surgery, the needle tip is continually alternating between states of occlusion and nonocclusion. This can create dramatic fluctuations in intraocular pressure, which could produce stress or traction on macular capillaries, choroidal vessels, vitreous, and other intraocular structures. Another alternative to increase infusion for sub-2-mm phaco is to pressurize the bottles with air pumps. The first air pump for cataract surgery was incorporated into the first prototype phacoemulsifier designed by Dr. Charles Kelman and Anton Banko. During the 1980s, a stand alone unit was offered by Greisharber (Schaffhausen, Switzerland) for anterior and posterior segment surgery. The current interest for the use of an air pump during cataract surgery was revived by Sunita Agarwal in 1999 to help in phakonit cataract surgery (Figure 6-1). Now the Stellaris (Bausch & Lomb, Aliso Viejo, CA) has inbuilt an air pump.

CHAMBER STABILITY

In designing the Stellaris for fluidics safety with 1.8-mm C-MICS, the decision was made to engineer each component of the system to work synergistically and optimize chamber stability without the need for excessively high or pressurized infusion bottles.

First, the C-MICS needle and sleeve were designed as a balanced pair using computational fluid dynamics, computer-aided design, and finite element analysis computer modeling. Various sizes and configurations were analyzed for their effects on intraocular pressure stability. The Stellaris Attune handpiece (Figure 6-2) was designed with a 50% larger infusion channel to deliver more BSS per second for any given bottle height (Figure 6-3).

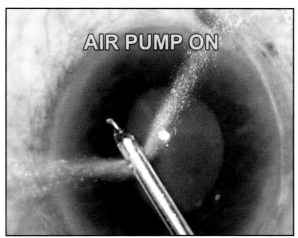

Figure 6-1. Air pump on (gas-forced infusion) in B-MICS (phakonit). Note the amount of fluid coming out of the irrigating chopper. (Photo courtesy of Dr. Agarwal's Group of Eye Hospitals and Eye Research Centre, Chennai, India.)[3]

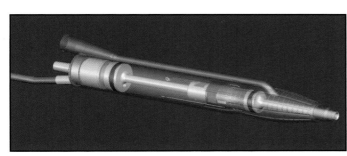

Figure 6-2. Stellaris Attune handpiece. (Reprinted with permission from Bausch & Lomb, Aliso Viejo, CA.)

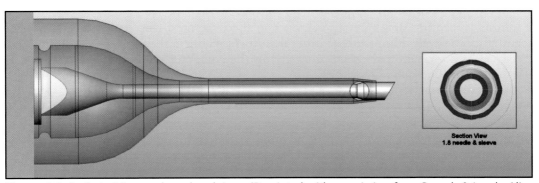

Figure 6-3. Stellaris 1.8-mm phaco handpiece. (Reprinted with permission from Bausch & Lomb, Aliso Viejo, CA.)

Stellaris tubing was created with a large diameter, high-compliance (soft) infusion line and a smaller diameter, low-compliance (stiff) aspiration line. This combination optimizes the ability to deliver BSS, stabilize the chamber, and minimize postocclusion surge for vacuum up to 300 mm Hg.

For higher C-MICS vacuum levels up to 600 mm Hg StableChamber (Bausch & Lomb) tubing was developed. This incorporates a short section of flexible tubing connecting the handpiece to a filter, and therefore maintains the natural flexibility and ergonomics of the standard tubing. The filter captures nucleus fragments and prevents clogging of the smaller and stiffer tubing that connects the filter to the console. This smaller internal diameter, very-low-compliance tubing increases resistance to outflow and further reduces the potential for chamber instability and postocclusion surge. The next step was the console.

Figure 6-4. Stellaris phaco machine. (Reprinted with permission from Bausch & Lomb, Aliso Viejo, CA.)

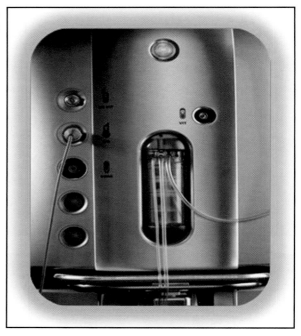

The Stellaris pump technology was completely redesigned and now incorporates a StableChamber Fluidics Module, which produces even more precise vacuum control than its predecessor, the venturi pump (Figure 6-4). It is electric and therefore has the additional advantage of eliminating the need for external compressed gas. The system uses 2 sensors to provide simultaneous feedback to the computer. One sensor directly monitors the speed of the pump and the other monitors vacuum at the aspiration cassette. The 2 sources of information are then processed by the computer's proportional-integral-differential (PID) computer algorithms.

PID algorithms are commonly used in jet aircraft control systems. In effect, the PID can compare the vacuum readings, updated every 5 ms, and analyze what has just occurred inside the cassette, what is happening now, and, in a sense, anticipate what may happen next. It can then feed back to control the pump speed and control a servo valve to modulate vacuum and pressure to further reduce postocclusion surge.

OPTIMIZING ULTRASONIC POWER

During phaco, as a surgeon steps down on the foot pedal to increase ultrasonic power, the actual effect is to increase the stroke or excursion of the needle. Stroke creates 4 major components of power: the acoustical wave, the mechanical impact of the tip (often referred to as the *jackhammer effect*), a fluid wave, and cavitation.

The acoustical wave is propelled in front of the tip at a velocity of approximately 1500 m per second at a frequency between 28.5 and 40 KHz depending on the manufacturer and can be directly visualized with a photographic technique called *shadow field photography*.[4] Its effect during phacoemulsification is poorly understood. It has, however, raised the question of why we can hear the handpiece during phaco if the frequency is ultrasonic. The sound we hear is from the mechanical vibrations and harmonic overtones generated by the ultrasonic vibration as well as cavitation from the hub of the needle.

The second component is the mechanical impact. As a phaco needle accelerates forward and strikes the nucleus, it can produce a cutting effect, sometimes referred to as the jackhammer effect. This impact may also tend to "push" the nucleus away from the needle tip, creating lens "chatter."

The third component, the fluid wave, is also created by the forward acceleration of the needle. As it pushes fluid from its leading edges, it adds to the tendency to drive nucleus away from the tip.

The fourth component of ultrasonic power is cavitation (Figure 6-5). As the phaco needle accelerates forward, it displaces fluid in front of it during what is called the *compression cycle*. As the needle retreats, a low-pressure area develops in front of the needle and cavitation bubbles begin to form during what is called the *expansion cycle*. As the needle moves forward again, it compresses the newly formed cavitation bubble, but because diffusion of gas (or vapor) into or out of the bubble is related to surface size, less gas can escape during compression and more gas can enter the bubble during expansion. Cavity growth during each expansion is, therefore, slightly larger than shrinkage during compression.

A cavitation bubble goes through a growth period of several cycles of expansion and contraction until it reaches a critical resonant size. Growing beyond this point, it can no longer absorb further energy and it implodes. During implosion, the cavitation bubble creates an unusual environment as it releases its energy in the form of heat, pressure, and microjets of fluid.

The heat is in excess of 5500°C (9000°F), hotter than the surface of the sun. The pressure waves are in excess of 1000 atmospheres (equivalent to being at the bottom of the ocean), and the fluid microjets have been photographed emanating from the imploding bubble and impacting the nearest hard surface at velocities of approximately 400 km per hour.

This raises the question of why cavitation does not damage the eye. The heat, pressure, and microjets from imploding cavitation bubbles occur in microscopic spaces in considerably less than a microsecond and have cooling rates above 10 billion degrees Celsius per second. At any given time, therefore, the bulk of the liquid remains at the ambient temperature.[5] Furthermore, with longitudinal (axial) phaco, studies have shown that cavitation is highly localized as a narrow beam of energy, less than 1 mm wide, directly in front of the tip. It should be noted that with torsional phaco, the cavitation bubbles are produced along the length of the needle shaft with little or no cavitation energy at the tip.[6] Possible effects of shaft cavitation in the incision should be considered if using torsional phaco without a sleeve for B-MICS.

In a separate experiment, Mark E. Schafer, PhD, used a hyperbaric chamber to study the relative cutting effects of the mechanical jackhammer energy and cavitation.[7] He designed the experiment with a standard phaco handpiece and needle suspended by a solenoid above a fixed-density resin block (approximately equivalent to a grade 3 nucleus).

With the hyperbaric chamber at normal atmospheric pressure and cavitation active, 20% power could burrow 5 mm into the block in less than 5 seconds. With the hyperbaric chamber pressurized, cavitation was suppressed, and at 20% power there was no effective cutting. By increasing the power to 60% with cavitation still suppressed, he could achieve 5 mm of cutting in approximately 10 seconds, but noted that it produced a "coring" effect and tended to clog the needle. This is consistent with the clinical recommendations of several OZil (Alcon, Fort Worth, TX) surgeons who recommend using longitudinal phaco along with torsional to prevent clogging. Based on this and other research, the current evidence suggests that the jackhammer effect initiates lens removal by cutting relatively large pieces of nucleus, which are then emulsified by cavitational energy.

Figure 6-5. Cavitation. (Photo courtesy of Dr. Terence Devine.)

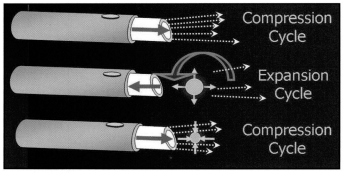

The Stellaris Attune handpiece was therefore designed with 6 crystals to expand the mechanical cutting by increasing its stroke 25%. It also optimizes cavitational emulsification by operating at a frequency of 28.5 KHz. It is known that the size and energy of cavitation bubbles are inversely proportional to the frequency creating them. At 28.5 KHz, the Attune handpiece produces cavitation bubbles of approximately 115 µm diameter compared to 82 µm with a 40-KHz machine. Cavitational energy is proportional to bubble volume. This means that bubbles formed at 28.5 KHz produce 2.68 times greater energy than those occurring at 40 KHz.

POWER MODULATION

All major manufacturers have incorporated various power modulation options with different trade names into their equipment. The concept was pioneered by Anton Banko, the co-inventor of phacoemulsification and founder of Surgical Design Corporation (Armonk, NY).

At the suggestion of Jerre Freeman, MD, Banko developed the first Pulser Power (Surgical Design, Armonk, NY), which allowed surgeons to choose from 1 to 20 pulses per second as an alternative to continuous power. Each pulse had an equal "on" period (pulse duration) and "off" period (pulse interval), creating a 50% duty cycle. The concept was that the off period would allow for aspiration flow and lens material to approach the needle tip unopposed by the jackhammer mechanical effect or the fluid wave and improve followability. The off period would also provide a time for cooling.

Since that original innovation, many refinements have been added, allowing surgeons choices in duty cycles, shorter on and off times (micropulses), and a variety of foot pedal options to control them such as burst, multiburst, fixed burst, and pulse modes.

The Stellaris was designed with the Attune Energy Management System (Bausch & Lomb), which allows on and off times as low as 2 ms, pulse rates up to 250 pps, and surgeon-programmable duty cycles. It offers a variety of power modes including pulse, burst, multiburst, fixed burst, and continuous power. It also offers a unique choice of traditional square wave pulses or waveform pulses. These names derive from their appearance on oscilloscope tracings.

WIRELESS, BLUETOOTH, DUAL LINEAR FOOT PEDAL

Another fluidics advance for the Stellaris is the wireless, Bluetooth, dual linear foot pedal. It has a variety of programmable options and can be used like a traditional phaco foot pedal in solely the up/down or pitch direction. In this case, the surgeon will program 2 or more low and high phaco settings and manually switch between them on the panel.

Most users, however, find a significant advantage in utilizing the dual linear function where power can be controlled in either the up and down pitch direction, or horizontally in the yaw direction. The vacuum can then be programmed to be controlled in the other direction. My personal preference for both standard phaco and C-MICS is to control linear power in the pitch direction and vacuum in the horizontal or yaw direction. This dual linear movement actually creates trilinear control.

For example, with C-MICS, using standard tubing, I program linear vacuum between 50 and 300 mm Hg in the yaw direction. As I step straight down in pitch to control linear power, I am generating 50 mm Hg, the low end of my linear vacuum range. If I then move my foot pedal horizontally in yaw, I will linearly increase vacuum. The further I move in yaw, the higher the vacuum will increase until I reach the horizontal limit of the foot pedal and the upper limit of my selected vacuum range.

To understand trilinear control, we need to recognize that if the phaco needle tip is not occluded, stepping straight down on the foot pedal produces 50 mm Hg vacuum in the collection cassette. Inside the eye, however, the effect is to create approximately 20 cc/min of flow with the C-MICS needle (larger needles would create higher flow for the same vacuum level).

Moving the foot pedal horizontally in the yaw direction will linearly increase the vacuum in the cassette, but in the eye we are increasing the flow and followability. With the foot pedal at full excursion in yaw, we reach our maximum selected vacuum level (in this example, 300 mm Hg). At that level, the flow inside the eye through the unoccluded C-MICS tip is approximately 45 cc/min. In other words, when the tip is not occluded, moving the foot pedal to the right increases the vacuum in the cassette, but inside the eye it is controlling the flow rate and providing linear followability.

Once the tip is occluded with nucleus, flow stops and vacuum migrates from the collection cassette to just inside the tip of the needle. Here it now provides vacuum holding force for chopping and aspiration. Moving the foot pedal horizontally in the yaw position is now controlling the vacuum holding force between 50 and 300 mm Hg.

The difference between a standard foot pedal and a dual linear foot pedal can be compared to the difference between driving a car with cruise control and using the gas pedal. On a straight highway where conditions are stable, cruise control is convenient. On a winding mountain road, however, the driver will need to speed up or slow down to match the changing conditions.

The dual linear foot pedal provides this gas pedal-like control of followability in the eye. We can use very low flow and followability when we are working close to iris or capsule and precisely increase the followability as we start to work more centrally in a safe position. This offers a level of safety and control not available with panel settings on a machine with a single-function foot pedal. This trilinear function facilitates phacoemulsification with any case using any technique but is particularly valuable when dealing with small pupils, IFIS cases with floppy iris, and cases with capsule tears or broken zonules.

StableChamber Tubing

For surgeons who prefer high vacuum techniques, 1.8-mm C-MICS can be safely performed up to 600 mm Hg with the StableChamber tubing.

StableChamber tubing incorporates a small internal diameter, low-compliance tubing for aspiration. This increases resistance to outflow and reduces the potential for chamber instability and postocclusion surge. Increased resistance to outflow also means that for any given vacuum level, there will be less flow and followability compared to standard tubing.

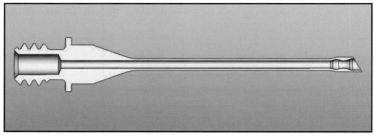

Figure 6-6. C-MICS phaco needle. (Reprinted with permission from Bausch & Lomb, Aliso Viejo, CA.)

Each surgeon may have a different preference for followability rates or how quickly or slowly material can be drawn to the phaco tip. My preference is 20 mL/min for sculpting for working close to capsule or iris and up to 45 cc/min to draw material to the tip when working centrally. With standard tubing, I achieve this flow range using a vacuum range of 50 to 300 mm Hg.

With StableChamber tubing, I can achieve that same flow range and followability by using a vacuum range of 200 to 600 mm Hg. With that setting, the "feel" for how slowly or quickly material is attracted to the tip is identical to the feel at the lower vacuum settings with standard tubing. The advantage of using 600 mm Hg with StableChamber tubing only becomes apparent when the tip is occluded.

At that time, flow stops and vacuum migrates to the tip, but instead of 300 mm Hg, there is 600 mm Hg vacuum holding force to facilitate chopping or quadrant removal.

1.8-MM COAXIAL MICROINCISIONAL CATARACT SURGERY TECHNIQUE

In terms of technique, C-MICS is compatible with any chopping, divide-and-conquer, phaco flip, or variation that a surgeon chooses (Figure 6-6). It should be stressed that proper incision size is important. The smaller infusion sleeves may be thinner and more easily crimped if the incision is too tight. Aside from crimping in the incision, they could also potentially crimp outside of the eye at the needle hub by "telescoping" as the surgeon advances the needle forward. This is not an issue with a true 1.8-mm incision, but surgeons should not "experiment" with smaller incisions with this technology.

There are 2 final points regarding the sleeves. The sleeve is designed for the infusion to be directed laterally at approximately 30 to 40 degrees through each of the infusion ports. If the sleeve is positioned too far back from the front "flair" of the needle, excess infusion will be directed forward, reducing followability and pushing lens material away from the tip.

The correct position is for the front edge of the sleeve to slightly overlap the wider front portion of the needle. Before entering the eye, the surgeon can verify this by engaging foot pedal position 1 (infusion) and observing that the majority of fluid is directed laterally.

The final point is that, with the smaller incision and somewhat thinner sleeve, it is easier to insert using reverse flow through the needle. This can be programmed to be activated by moving the foot pedal to the left in yaw. The reverse flow immediately inflates and lubricates the corneal tunnel and pressurizes the anterior chamber before the sleeve is introduced.

SUMMARY

The Stellaris was engineered to balance multiple technologies to optimize safety and efficiency for 1.8-mm C-MICS and B-MICS. This integrated design offers these same advantages for traditional 2.8-mm techniques and can readily be adapted to go below 1.8 mm for C-MICS as lens technology and surgeon preferences evolve.

REFERENCES

1. Agarwal A, Agarwal S, Agarwal A. Phakonit: a new technique of removing cataracts through a 0.9 mm incision. In: Agarwal A, Agarwal S, Agarwal A, eds. *Phacoemulsification, Laser Cataract Surgery and Foldable IOLs*. New Delhi, India: Jaypee; 1998:139-143.
2. Agarwal A, Agarwal S, Agarwal A, Narang P, Narang S. Phakonit: phacoemulsification through a 0.9 mm corneal incision. *J Cataract Refract Surg.* 2001;27(10):1548-1552.
3. Agarwal A. *Bimanual Phaco: Mastering the Phakonit/MICS Technique*. Thorofare, NJ: Slack Incorporated; 2004.
4. Brown B, Goodman J. *High-Intensity Ultrasonics*. Princeton, NJ: London Iliffe Books Ltd.; 1965:40.
5. Suslick KS. The chemical effects of ultrasound. *Sci Am.* 1989;260:80-86.
6. Schafer ME. In vitro and ex vivo measurements of cavitation from ultrasonic phacoemulsification systems. Paper presented at: ASCRS Annual Meeting: Washington DC; April 15-20, 2005.
7. Schafer ME. Quantifying the impact of cavitation in decreasing the use of ultrasonic energy during phacoemulsification. Paper presented at: ASCRS Annual Meeting: San Francisco, CA; March 17-22, 2006.

CHAPTER 7

MICS AND THE ABBOTT MEDICAL OPTICS PLATFORM

George H. H. Beiko, BM, BCh (Oxon), FRCSC

Microincisional cataract surgery (MICS)[1,2] would not be possible at all without the considerable advancements in ultrasound power modulation first introduced with the WhiteStar Sovereign phaco system (Abbot Medical Optics [AMO], Santa Ana, CA).

WHITESTAR MICROPULSE TECHNOLOGY

The first-generation phacoemulsification machines employed continuous 100% ultrasound power. The first innovation was the advent of the foot pedal, which allowed for linear control of the power, but this was still delivered in a continuous fashion.

To understand the subsequent innovations, some definitions must be reviewed. *Pulse mode* refers to the energy being delivered for a period of time followed by a rest period. The on and rest periods are of equal duration. For example, a setting of 4 pulses per second (pps) represents a pulse of 125 ms followed by a rest of 125 ms; thus, each cycle is 250 ms. In pulse mode, the foot pedal controls the amount of power. *Burst mode* results in a preset amount of energy being delivered; depression of the foot pedal determines the number of bursts per unit time.

A *duty cycle* consists of a period of energy delivery followed by an energy-free or rest period. The duty cycle refers to the percentage of time that ultrasound is on; it is calculated by dividing the amount of time that ultrasound is on by the total time of on and off periods. Thus, continuous ultrasound has a duty cycle of 100%, whereas conventional phaco has a duty cycle of 50%.

The primary impediment to bare-needle MICS with continuous phacoemulsification was the potential for wound burn. Continuous phaco with a bare needle results in friction between the needle and the wound; an increase in wound temperature and collagen coagulation leading to wound burn; and consequences including wound distortion, wound leak, and induced corneal astigmatism.

The introduction of WhiteStar cold phaco technology in 2001 for the AMO Sovereign phacoemulsification system allowed for programmable pulse and rest durations. This technology made it possible to vary the duration of the pulse and the rest period independently. Pulses and rests as short as 4 ms could be utilized, and the ultrasound on/off cycle could occur at two-tenths of a millisecond. An example is a 33% duty cycle with 6 ms of applied energy followed by 12 ms of rest period that results in 55 pps.

By increasing the rest period and decreasing the pulse period, fluid flowing from the irrigation handpiece to the phaco tip in bimanual MICS (B-MICS) effectively increases the amount of time that a nuclear fragment is in contact with the phaco tip. Thus, a low duty cycle (increased rest period) facilitates holding of the nuclear fragment.

Increasing the energy period and decreasing the rest period (high duty cycle) in contrast results in better cutting of the cataract. Corneal wound burn will occur at a temperature of 60°C and can occur at lower temperatures of 45°C if the temperature is sustained.[3] With WhiteStar technology, Steinert and Schafer showed that WhiteStar's micro- or hyperpulsing reduced the temperature rise at the phaco tip by as much as 20°C.[4] Laboratory studies demonstrated that the maximum wound temperature using WhiteStar ranged from 21 to 37°C,[3,5,6] well below the 45 to 50°C threshold for thermal collagen damage. In fact, the energy needed to obtain a wound burn during bimanual phaco with a bare aspiration needle in human cadaver eyes was extremely high—well beyond anything one would see in a normal clinical setting.[3] Donnenfeld and colleagues provided confirmation of this in a clinical study in which temperature gradients, measured directly adjacent to the wound in 10 patients undergoing MICS, never exceeded 34°C.[7]

Taken together, these studies showed that the phaco sleeve was superfluous and that microincisional phaco with a bare needle could be safely performed in human eyes.

WhiteStar micropulsing enables a surgeon to employ variable pulse-to-rest ratios; the duration of the pulse and the rest can be programmed for a set time in the duty cycle. In this author's experience, the micropulse period is set for 4, 6, or 8 ms and the rest period for 4, 8, 12, or 24 ms. The duty cycle consists of combinations of these microbursts and rests, depending on whether the goal is emulsification or attraction of the nuclear fragments. Figure 7-1 illustrates the comparison between continuous power, traditional pulse, and micropulse with a 1:2 duty cycle ratio.

Earlier pulse/burst modes allowed some modulation of continuous-wave phaco energy, controlled by the surgeon with the foot pedal. But these were not as effective as WhiteStar in allowing safe MICS.[8,9] The automated rapid ultrasound pulsing in WhiteStar functions much like a fluorescent lightbulb, with the rapid on/off cycling allowing the phaco tip to stay cold. This technology reduced the total energy into the eye by 50% to 70%.[10]

Moreover, the reduction in energy was accomplished without sacrificing cutting efficiency. Several studies demonstrated that even very hard nuclei (3+ and harder) could be safely and effectively removed through microincisions using the WhiteStar system.[9,11,12] Later, performance in hard nuclei was further improved with Variable WhiteStar, which permitted the surgeon to adjust the duty cycle based on the cutting requirements of the case.

In addition to virtually eliminating the risk of thermal damage, WhiteStar micropulse technology has had other benefits as well. Because it is more efficient and requires less ultrasound energy, the effective phaco time (EPT) is shorter, turbulence and chatter of nuclear material in the eye is limited, and trauma to the trabecular meshwork and endothelium is reduced. Less damage to the trabecular meshwork minimizes postoperative intraocular pressure spikes.[13] Less endothelial damage results in less endothelial cell loss.

WhiteStar pulsing draws nuclear fragments to the phaco tip, optimizing transient cavitational energy (which produces a momentary water jet that breaks up nuclear fragments through high-energy, localized implosions) and minimizing stable cavitational energy (vibration of cavitation bubbles that has no effect on nuclear material). Maximizing selective transient cavitational energy and minimizing stable cavitational energy optimizes cutting performance and reduces overall energy input and heat production at the wound.

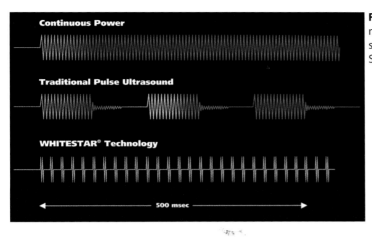

Figure 7-1. Comparison of energy modes. (Reprinted with permission from Abbott Medical Optics, Santa Ana, CA.)

When researchers compared turbulence with and without WhiteStar using high-resolution color digital ultrasound imaging, increased fluid velocity away from the phaco tip as continuous phaco power increased was demonstrated, whereas the amount of such turbulence with WhiteStar was much more limited (Figure 7-2).[4] This explains why conventional phaco pushes away nuclear fragments and accounts for the better followability reported with WhiteStar. High-speed digital photography also showed that the brief rest periods in WhiteStar's on/off pulses diminished the repelling force of the vibrating phaco tip, reducing chatter and turbulence.[14] For patients, the result may be a healthier endothelium. Fishkind and colleagues reported less endothelial cell loss at 3 months with WhiteStar compared to standard Sovereign phaco (319.6 versus 430.3 cells/mm^2).[15]

With previous phaco systems, when phacoemulsification of a nuclear fragment resulted in an occlusion break, there was a transient inability of flow to keep up with vacuum, the intraocular pressure in the anterior chamber dropped, and the chamber shallowed; this is the phenomenom of *surge*. The other innovation with WhiteStar for the Sovereign system was surge control via "smart pump" strategy; this relies on sensors that measure the vacuum 50 times per second. When the phaco tip is occluded, the vacuum rises to half of the preset value and aspiration flow decreases slowly to 0 mL/min. This strategy avoids the momentary overaspiration that occurs with postocclusion surge. Minimizing surge minimizes complications of posterior capsular rupture and phaco-induced iris damage.

Variable WhiteStar

The introduction of Variable WhiteStar allows a surgeon to have linear control of WhiteStar energy delivery. With this software, a surgeon can choose and tailor the WhiteStar duty cycles. Up to 4 duty cycles can be programmed into position 3 on the foot pedal; depression of the foot pedal allows for linear progression through these cycles. Thus, each phaco setting can have increased flexibility because there is the potential to have 4 duty cycles available in foot pedal position 3, allowing a surgeon to maneuver through various densities of nuclear fragments to optimize the delivery of energy to the cataract and to maintain followability (Figure 7-3).

WhiteStar ICE

Several additional features were introduced with the second-generation micropulse technology for Sovereign. WhiteStar ICE (increased control and efficiency) included the

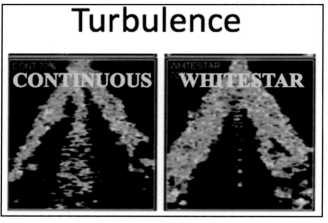

Figure 7-2. Experimental simulation of turbulence, comparing WhiteStar to continuous phaco. Continous phaco has increased fluid velocity away from the phaco tip, resulting in a repulsion of the nuclear fragments.[4]

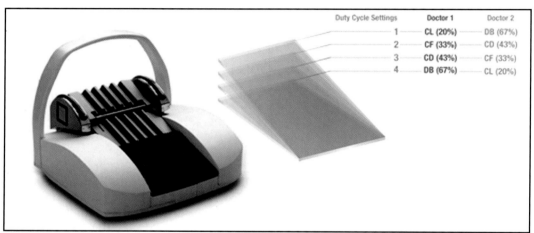

Figure 7-3. An example of Variable WhiteStar settings in foot position 3. This software allows programming of up to 4 duty cycles and the amount of up/down excursion of the foot pedal for each duty cycle. (Reprinted with permission from Abbott Medical Optics, Santa Ana, CA.)

foot pedal–controlled variable-duty cycles mentioned above for better efficacy in hard nuclei, advanced pulse shaping, and an automated chamber stabilization algorithm known as chamber automated stabilization environment (CASE).

The pulse shaping is probably the best-known feature of WhiteStar ICE. Engineers added a microburst at the beginning of each pulse to maximize cavitational energy (Figure 7-4). The microburst physically separates the nuclear material from the phaco tip, allowing the creation of a microvoid between the occluded tip and the nuclear material. Fresh balanced salt solution can get into the microvoid, between the tip and the nuclear material, where it interacts with the ultrasound power to accelerate cavitational emulsification and increase the ultrasound efficiency (Figure 7-5). The pulse amplitude can be customized to increase, decrease, or remain steady throughout the phaco procedure (Figure 7-6).

WhiteStar ICE pulse shaping reduced EPT. Dewey reported that his EPT with ICE for a 3+ cataract was down from 4.63 to 3.70 s—about a 20% reduction.[16] ICE prevents full occlusion but keeps the nuclear particle adjacent to the tip for magnetic followability. This reduced the surgeon's reliance on mechanical manipulation in the eye, paralleling the accomplishments with MICS. With the flow directed from the other side of the chamber in a B-MICS procedure, the surgeon has tremendous control over nuclear fragments.

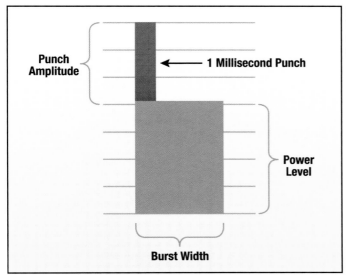

Figure 7-4. ICE pulse created by WhiteStar ICE technology. (Reprinted with permission from Abbott Medical Optics, Santa Ana, CA.)

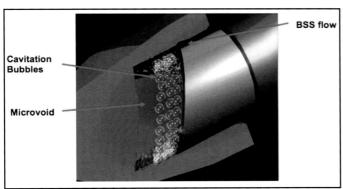

Figure 7-5. Artist rendering of ICE pulse. (Reprinted with permission from Abbott Medical Optics, Santa Ana, CA.)

CHAMBER AUTOMATED STABILIZATION ENVIRONMENT

Of the WhiteStar ICE advances, CASE was probably the most important, as it dramatically increases safety and enhances the role of fluidics in phacoemulsification. CASE dramatically reduces surge. Prior to CASE, the power modulation or occlusion modes of various phaco systems were only able to regulate the rising portion of the vacuum curve. CASE significantly reduces postocclusion surge by automating control of the descending vacuum curve, where the sudden drop in vacuum is most likely to break the posterior capsule. CASE constantly monitors the anterior chamber, begins to recognize occlusion even before it happens (when vacuum levels have crossed a predetermined "up threshold"), and then proactively reverses the pump to step down the vacuum to predetermined levels before the occlusion break occurs (Figure 7-7). This essentially duplicates what an experienced surgeon might be able to do with the foot pedal, but does it much faster (within 26 ms of the occlusion with previous versions of WhiteStar; down to just 20 ms with CASE).

According to some reports, CASE reduces surge by 56% (Figure 7-8). Regardless of the surgeon's preferred technique (MICS or standard coaxial) and instrumentation, this technology improves the safety of phaco by maintaining an extremely stable chamber.

SIGNATURE SYSTEM

The latest-generation phacoemulsification system from AMO is the WhiteStar Signature system with Fusion Fluidics. Existing technology has been strengthened in this system and a number of key innovations have been added.

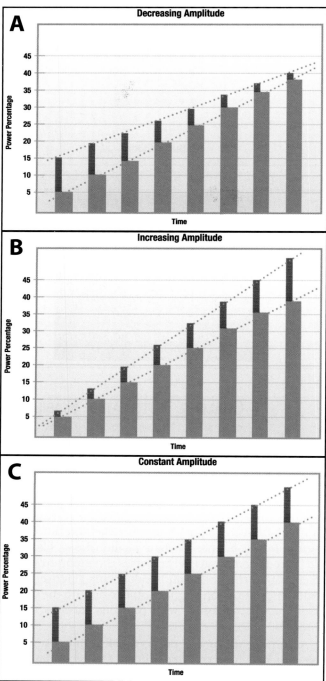

Figure 7-6. The amplitude of the ICE pulse can be increased, decreased, or maintained at a constant level, depending on surgeon preference. (Reprinted with permission from Abbott Medical Optics, Santa Ana, CA.)

MICS AND THE ABBOTT MEDICAL OPTICS PLATFORM

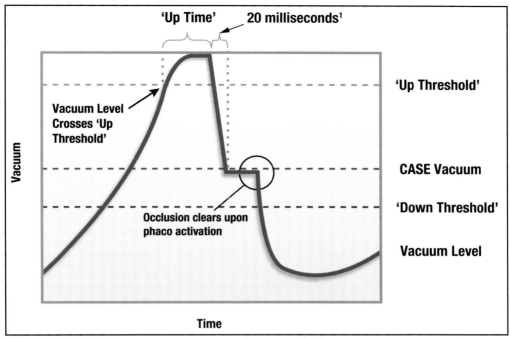

Figure 7-7. WhiteStar Signature system with Fusion Fluidics Proactive Vacuum Adjustment. (Reprinted with permission from Abbott Medical Optics, Santa Ana, CA.)

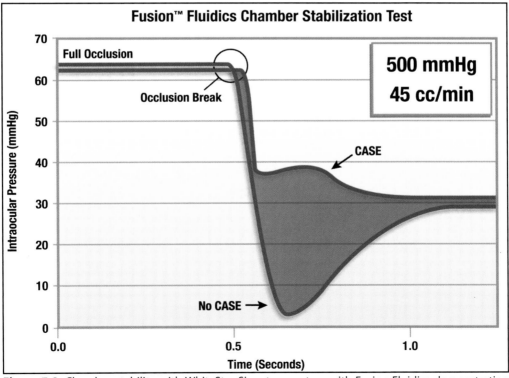

Figure 7-8. Chamber stability with WhiteStar Signature system with Fusion Fluidics demonstrating approximately 56% less surge with a 20-guage tip. (Reprinted with permission from Abbott Medical Optics, Santa Ana, CA.)

77

Fusion Fluidics encompasses both the CASE vacuum-regulating algorithms as well as automated adjustments to the aspiration rate and phaco power/mode settings. Reaction time to pre-occlusion vacuum "up time" is even faster, as noted previously. And for the first time, rise—the speed at which the pump stops and starts—can be controlled as an independent variable. Surgeons can adjust rise time according to their own technique and the hardness of the nucleus in a particular case, further enhancing surgeon comfort and chamber stability.

In MICS cases, the separation of flow and vacuum increases one's flexibility to primarily use the fluidics to remove soft nuclei with minimal or no ultrasound power at all. The peristaltic pump is also more powerful, which helps to compensate for any disadvantages of a smaller phaco tip for MICS. There is a 20% increase in the peristaltic flow rate, up to 60 cc/min, and a 30% increase in peristaltic vacuum, up to a maximum of 650 mm Hg. CASE is really a prerequisite to use these higher parameters safely.

The Signature system is an extremely stable platform with considerable advantages. When tested against other manufacturers' devices, Signature had both the lowest postocclusion surge and the lowest unoccluded flow vacuum.[17,18]

DUAL-PUMP TECHNOLOGY

In addition to its advanced peristaltic pump with all of the Fusion Fluidics features, AMO Signature also has a high-quality Venturi pump. For the first time, surgeons can switch on the fly between peristaltic and Venturi pumps and the system can be preprogrammed to switch between pumps as needed within a given procedure.

Venturi pumps are more powerful and more reliable in low-vacuum situations, whereas peristaltic pumps have typically offered greater control and safety for anterior segment surgery. There are few data thus far on the advantages of one pump style versus another for MICS. In a recent study from Turkey, the authors found that a Venturi pump significantly shortened the surgery time in B-MICS cases.[19]

Dual-pump technology has the added advantages of enabling a surgeon to use the Venturi high-vacuum performance and holding power, if desired, and the flexibility of both modalities for multi-surgeon environments where preferences may vary from surgeon to surgeon.

ELLIPS

Nonlongitudinal phaco modes are another important innovation in cataract surgery. Alcon's OZil (Fort Worth, TX) torsional phaco handpiece for the Alcon INFINITI system was the first to add a horizontal direction to the in-and-out motion of longitudinal phaco. AMO's version, Ellips Transversal Phaco, was introduced in 2008. With this handpiece, the needle moves simultaneously in an elliptical and longitudinal pattern, making it the first technology to simultaneously blend longitudinal and nonlongitudinal modes and the first that can be used with a straight-tip needle.

Ellips transversal phaco offers increased cutting power, especially in brunescent nuclei, because it is constantly emulsifying in all directions (Figure 7-9). It also reduces the amount of energy in the eye. These modes are the least likely of any phaco technique to cause a wound burn, so they make sleeveless MICS even safer to contemplate. Finally, the transversal mode limits the jackhammering action of longitudinal phaco, thereby enhancing followability. This may also make MICS easier to perform through small incisions with smaller instrumentation.

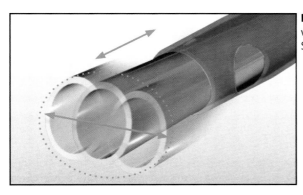

Figure 7-9. Ellips transversal phaco. (Reprinted with permission from Abbott Medical Optics, Santa Ana, CA.)

All in all, the Signature system greatly reduces the surgeon's anxiety level by reducing routine trauma, endothelial cell loss, and chamber shallowing, as well as greatly reducing the risk of capsular rupture and vitrectomy. It permits great customization and individualization for the surgeon's preferred techniques and parameters, including for complex or challenging cases.

These benefits accrue regardless of whether one chooses to perform standard coaxial phaco or B-MICS, but they make MICS much more efficient and safe. Moreover, the Signature's advanced Surgical Media Center, though perhaps not critical to the surgery itself, facilitates learning new techniques such as MICS.

Personal Technique

ANESTHESIA

I routinely use topical anesthesia for all of my cases. I have used 0.75% bupivacaine, amethocaine, and lidocaine gel with comparable efficacy. I currently use a lidocaine gel preparation—the mixture is formulated by the clinic pharmacy and consists of 5 mL 2% xylocaine (20 mg/mL) and 4 drops each of 10% epinephrine, 1% cyclopentolate, 1% tropicamide, ofloxacin (Ocuflox), and ketorolac ophthalmic (Acular).[20] The mixture is administered 0.3 mL via a tuberculin (TB) syringe, 1 hour and 10 min preop.

Intraoperatively, I use 1% unpreserved xylocaine to hydrodissect and/or hydrodelineate the nucleus. This provides additional anesthesia to the ciliary body; it also may decrease posterior capsule opacification (PCO) (personal communication, Professor Rupert Menapace, 2005).

INCISIONS

I routinely sit at the head of the patient for both right and left eyes. I place my incisions at the 10 and 2 o'clock positions. The incisions are as small as possible so as to prevent leakage of irrigating fluid through these wounds during implementation of instruments. Preventing leakage ensures a stable chamber. I employ a trapezoidal blade; the goal is to make the internal opening smaller than the external, so as to minimize oar-locking. Since I use 19-gauge irrigating and phaco tips, I use a blade design of 1.2 > 1.4 mm.

I prefer a diamond blade because of the increased control in incision construction; however, I do use metal blades in one of the surgical centers without significant problems.

In order to minimize astigmatic induction, I make a 3-plane, Langerman's type of incision at the 10 o'clock position. The initial groove is in the posterior limbus, through conjunctiva, but as anterior as possible. This groove is longer than the wound so as to minimize conjunctival ballooning. I make the incision in the posterior limbus as I prefer to have conjunctival covering of the incision so as to promote a faster seal of the incision and decrease the risk of endopthalmitis. The entry into the anterior chamber with the 1.2 > 1.4 mm trapezoidal blade is made through this incision with a tunnel of 1.5 to 2.0 mm. Following phacoemulsification and cortical cleanup, this incision is enlarged to 2.8 mm for IOL insertion.

I make a Wong pocket anterior to the 10 o'clock incision. This pocket is hydrated at the end of the cataract surgery so as to seal the wound more effectively. I use balanced salt solution (BSS) to hydrate, but see no objection to using steroid or antibiotics, as advocated by some authors who believe these drugs act as a reservoir.

The incision at the 2 o'clock position, also made with the 1.2 > 1.4 mm trapezoidal blade, is a 2-plane incision without the benefit of a groove, also in the posterior limbus. No groove is made as this incision is not enlarged.

INSTRUMENTS

I use a 19-gauge straight phaco tip with a 300 bevel. I use the phaco tip with the bevel down for phacoemulsification. This tip is introduced through the 10 o'clock incision.

The irrigating hand piece is a straight 19-gauge cannula with a Sinskey hook at the tip. The tip also has 2 side ports for irrigation. This device is custom made for me by Katena (Denville, NJ). I find it is versatile as the round Sinskey tip allows me not only to manipulate and chop the nucleus, but also to be able to touch delicate tissues such as the iris or capsule. This is used at the 2 o'clock incision.

I use a microforceps for capsulorrhexis creation. Any number of instrument companies currently make these, with a 23-gauge design for easy manipulation through the small incisions employed in bimanual MICS. My preference is for the Fine/Hoffman Capsulorrhexis forceps with Seibel Rhexis Ruler (MicroSurgical Technology, Redmond, WA) as this device allows for accurate rhexis sizing—something that is becoming a critical issue in some premium IOL implantation.

I also use the Akahoshi Combo prechopper (Asico, Westmont, IL) in the majority of my cases. In 1 to 3+ nuclear sclerosis cases, I employ it directly to break up the nucleus into either 4 quadrants (if there is easy rotation of the hydrodissected nucleus) or 3 segments with a "V" configuration if the nucleus is difficult to rotate. I have found that this device reduces the amount of phaco energy by 45% in my cases. In 4+ or brunescent cataracts, I will phaco a central groove, making it so deep that the red reflex begins to come through. I will then place the prechopper into the groove and separate the halves of the nucleus with minimal force and manipulation; I find that this strategy even works with the dense leathery cataracts.

OPHTHALMIC VISCOSURGICAL DEVICES (OVDS)

I use sodium hyaluronate (Healon 5) in all of my cases. For capsulorrhexis creation, I will inject enough Healon 5 to block the incision at the 10 o'clock position. Typically, I will fill the chamber half full with viscoelastic, using the viscoelastic to tamponade the anterior capsule. The remainder of the chamber will be BSS.

Healon 5 is used to manipulate the tissues in the eye. The pupil is enlarged with this OVD, and is particularly useful for floppy iris cases or cases where there has been damage to the iris. Healon 5 also can be useful for tissue separation, such as cases of anterior or posterior synechiae.

I find that the Healon 5 provides excellent control for capsulorrhexis creation, as the leading flap remains in the position it is placed. Capsulorrhexis microforceps are used to create the capsulorrhexis.

See Table 7-1 for my personal bimanual settings with WhiteStar software.

Table 7-1

BIMANUAL SETTINGS FOR DR. BEIKO
INCORPORATING VARIABLE WHITESTAR SOFTWARE

Software Version   Version 2.033
Surgeon   Dr. Beiko
Program   Bi-Manual
Date   28.02.2008 / 03:00:22 PM

PHACO 1—Soft Nuclei

Active	YES
Occluded Mode	Off
Case Mode	Off
Pump Type	Peristaltic
Bottle Height	66 cm

Unoccluded Settings

Aspiration	10 cc/min Panel
Vacuum	200 mmHg Linear
Power	10% Linear
Mode	Continuous
Pump Ramp	70
WS	6/12 (33%, 55 pps)

WS Settings

Continuous	6/12 (33%, 55 pps)
Variable WS 1	
FootPedal Position 3	0-25%—6/24 (20%, 33 pps)
FootPedal Position 3	26-50%—6/12 (33%, 55 pps)
FootPedal Position 3	51-75%—6/8 (43%, 71 pps)
FootPedal Position 3	76-100%—8/4 (67%, 83 pps)
Variable WS 2	
FootPedal Position 3	0-25%—8/4 (67%, 83 pps)
FootPedal Position 3	26-50%—6/8 (43%, 71 pps)
FootPedal Position 3	51-75%—6/12 (33%, 55 pps)
FootPedal Position 3	76-100%—6/24 (20%, 33 pps)

Pulse Shaping Settings

Active	NO
% Kick: Low End Range	5
% Kick: High End of Range	5
Low Power Limit	0
High Power Limit	80

Occlusion Mode Settings

Aspiration	18 cc/min
Vacuum	25 mmHg
Power	40% Linear
Mode	Continuous
Pump Ramp	85
WS	6/12 (33%, 55 pps)

WS Settings

Continuous	6/12 (33%, 55 pps)
Variable WS 1	
FootPedal Position 3	0-25%—6/24 (20%, 33 pps)
FootPedal Position 3	26-50%—6/12 (33%, 55 pps)
FootPedal Position 3	51-75%—6/8 (43%, 71 pps)
FootPedal Position 3	76-100%—8/4 (67%, 83 pps)
Variable WS 2	
FootPedal Position 3	0-25%—8/4 (67%, 83 pps)
FootPedal Position 3	26-50%—6/8 (43%, 71 pps)
FootPedal Position 3	51-75%—6/12 (33%, 55 pps)
FootPedal Position 3	76-100%—6/24 (20%, 33 pps)

Pulse Shaping Settings

Active	NO
% Kick: Low End Range	5
% Kick: High End of Range	5
Low Power Limit	0
High Power Limit	80

Case Mode Settings

Down Threshold	70 mmHg
CASE Vacuum	85 mmHg
Up Threshold	100 mmHg
Up Time	300 mSec
One Touch	Standard

PHACO 2—Standard Nuclei (up to 3+)

Active	YES
Occluded Mode	On
Case Mode	Off
Pump Type	Peristaltic
Bottle Height	76 cm

Unoccluded Settings

Aspiration	22 cc/min Panel
Vacuum	250 mmHg Linear
Power	10% Linear
Mode	Continuous
Pump Ramp	65
WS	Variable WS 1

Table 7-1 (continued)

WS Settings

Continuous	6/12 (33%, 55 pps)
Variable WS 1	
FootPedal Position 3	0-25%—6/24 (20%, 33 pps)
FootPedal Position 3	26-50%—6/24 (20%, 33 pps)
FootPedal Position 3	51-75%—4/8 (33%, 83 pps)
FootPedal Position 3	76-100%—6/8 (43%, 71 pps)
Variable WS 2	
FootPedal Position 3	0-25%—8/4 (67%, 83 pps)
FootPedal Position 3	26-50%—6/8 (43%, 71 pps)
FootPedal Position 3	51-75%—6/12 (33%, 55 pps)
FootPedal Position 3	76-100%—6/24 (20%, 33 pps)

Pulse Shaping Settings

Active	YES
% Kick: Low End Range	10
% Kick: High End of Range	10
Low Power Limit	0
High Power Limit	80

Occlusion Mode Settings

Aspiration	20 cc/min
Vacuum	200 mmHg
Power	15% Linear
Mode	Continuous
Pump Ramp	65
WS	Variable WS 1

WS Settings

Continuous	6/12 (33%, 55 pps)
Variable WS 1	
FootPedal Position 3	0-25%—6/24 (20%, 33 pps)
FootPedal Position 3	26-50%—6/24 (20%, 33 pps)
FootPedal Position 3	51-75%—4/8 (33%, 83 pps)
FootPedal Position 3	76-100%—6/8 (43%, 71 pps)
Variable WS 2	
FootPedal Position 3	0-25%—8/4 (67%, 83 pps)
FootPedal Position 3	26-50%—6/8 (43%, 71 pps)
FootPedal Position 3	51-75%—6/12 (33%, 55 pps)
FootPedal Position 3	76-100%—6/24 (20%, 33 pps)

Pulse Shaping Settings

Active	YES
% Kick: Low End Range	10
% Kick: High End of Range	10
Low Power Limit	0
High Power Limit	80

Case Mode Settings

Down Threshold	109 mmHg
CASE Vacuum	144 mmHg
Up Threshold	176 mmHg
Up Time	1020 mSec
One Touch	Standard

PHACO 3—HARD NUCLEI (3-4+)

Active	YES
Occluded Mode	On
Case Mode	On
Pump Type	Peristaltic
Bottle Height	76 cm

Unoccluded Settings

Aspiration	22 cc/min Panel
Vacuum	300 mmHg Linear
Power	35% Linear
Mode	Continuous
Pump Ramp	65
WS	Variable WS 1

WS Settings

Continuous	6/12 (33%, 55 pps)
Variable WS 1	
FootPedal Position 3	0-25%—6/24 (20%, 33 pps)
FootPedal Position 3	26-50%—6/12 (33%, 55 pps)
FootPedal Position 3	51-75%—6/8 (43%, 71 pps)
FootPedal Position 3	76-100%—6/8 (43%, 71 pps)
Variable WS 2	
FootPedal Position 3	0-25%—4/8 (33%, 83 pps)
FootPedal Position 3	26-50%—4/8 (33%, 83 pps)
FootPedal Position 3	51-75%—6/8 (43%, 71 pps)
FootPedal Position 3	76-100%—8/4 (67%, 83 pps)

Pulse Shaping Settings

Active	YES
% Kick: Low End Range	10
% Kick: High End of Range	10
Low Power Limit	0
High Power Limit	80

Occlusion Mode Settings

Aspiration	24 cc/min
Vacuum	150 mmHg
Power	50% Linear
Mode	Continuous
Pump Ramp	65
WS	Variable WS 2

Table 7-1 (continued)

WS Settings		**Variable WS 2**	
Continuous	6/12 (33%, 55 pps)	FootPedal Position 3	0-25%—8/4 (67%, 83 pps)
Variable WS 1		FootPedal Position 3	26-50%—6/8 (43%, 71 pps)
FootPedal Position 3	0-25%—6/24 (20%, 33 pps)	FootPedal Position 3	51-75%—6/12 (33%, 55 pps)
FootPedal Position 3	26-50%—6/12 (33%, 55 pps)	FootPedal Position 3	76-100%—6/24 (20%, 33 pps)
FootPedal Position 3	51-75%—6/8 (43%, 71 pps)	**Pulse Shaping Settings**	
FootPedal Position 3	76-100%—8/4 (67%, 83 pps)	Active	NO
Variable WS 2		% Kick: Low End Range	5
FootPedal Position 3	0-25%—8/4 (67%, 83 pps)	% Kick: High End of Range	5
FootPedal Position 3	26-50%—6/8 (43%, 71 pps)	Low Power Limit	0
FootPedal Position 3	51-75%—6/12 (33%, 55 pps)	High Power Limit	80
FootPedal Position 3	76-100%—6/24 (20%, 33 pps)	**Occlusion Mode Settings**	
Pulse Shaping Settings		Aspiration	24 cc/min
Active	YES	Vacuum	30 mmHg
% Kick: Low End Range	10	Power	40% Linear
% Kick: High End of Range	10	Mode	Continuous
Low Power Limit	0	Pump Ramp	85
High Power Limit	80	WS	6/12 (33%, 55 pps)
Case Mode Settings		**WS Settings**	
Down Threshold	200 mmHg	Continuous	6/12 (33%, 55 pps)
CASE Vacuum	235 mmHg	Variable WS 1	
Up Threshold	270 mmHg	FootPedal Position 3	0-25%—6/24 (20%, 33 pps)
Up Time	1060 mSec	FootPedal Position 3	26-50%—6/12 (33%, 55 pps)
One Touch	Standard	FootPedal Position 3	51-75%—6/8 (43%, 71 pps)
PHACO 4—Brunescent Cataract		FootPedal Position 3	76-100%—8/4 (67%, 83 pps)
Active	YES	Variable WS 2	
Occluded Mode	Off	FootPedal Position 3	0-25%—8/4 (67%, 83 pps)
Case Mode	Off	FootPedal Position 3	26-50%—6/8 (43%, 71 pps)
Pump Type	Peristaltic	FootPedal Position 3	51-75%—6/12 (33%, 55 pps)
Bottle Height	76 cm	FootPedal Position 3	76-100%—6/24 (20%, 33 pps)
Unoccluded Settings		**Pulse Shaping Settings**	
Aspiration	20 cc/min Panel	Active	NO
Vacuum	30 mmHg Linear	% Kick: Low End Range	5
Power	45% Linear	% Kick: High End of Range	5
Mode	Continuous	Low Power Limit	0
Pump Ramp	70	High Power Limit	80
WS	6/8 (43%, 71 pps)	**Case Mode Settings**	
WS Settings		Down Threshold	200 mmHg
Continuous	6/8 (43%, 71 pps)	CASE Vacuum	250 mmHg
Variable WS 1		Up Threshold	300 mmHg
FootPedal Position 3	0-25%—6/24 (20%, 33 pps)	Up Time	300 mSec
FootPedal Position 3	26-50%—6/12 (33%, 55 pps)	One Touch	Standard
FootPedal Position 3	51-75%—6/8 (43%, 71 pps)		
FootPedal Position 3	76-100%—8/4 (67%, 83 pps)		

Table 7-1 (continued)

IA 1
Active	YES
Aspiration	30 cc/min Panel
Vacuum	300 mmHg Linear
Pump Type	Peristaltic
Bottle Height	43 cm
Pump Ramp	80

IA 2
Active	YES
Aspiration	6 cc/min Linear
Vacuum	10 mmHg Panel
Pump Type	Peristaltic
Bottle Height	50 cm
Pump Ramp	80

IA 3
Active	YES
Aspiration	40 cc/min Linear
Vacuum	500 mmHg Panel
Pump Type	Peristaltic
Bottle Height	50 cm
Pump Ramp	80

VIT 1
Active	YES
Aspiration	30 cc/min Panel
Vacuum	300 mmHg Panel
CUT	800 IAC, Panel
Pump Type	Peristaltic
Bottle Height	30 cm
Pump Ramp	100

VIT 2
Active	YES
Aspiration	12 cc/min Panel
Vacuum	225 mmHg Panel
CUT	450 IAC, Linear
Pump Type	Peristaltic
Bottle Height	30 cm
Pump Ramp	100

DIA 1
Active	YES
Power	30 Linear

DIA 2
Active	YES
Power	30 Burst

Footpedal Settings

PHACO
Switch Right	Next Sub Mode
Switch Left	Previous Sub Mode
Switch Config1	Off
Switch Config2	Next Major Mode

IA
Switch Right	Next Sub Mode
Switch Left	Previous Sub Mode
Switch Config1	Off
Switch Config2	Next Major Mode

VIT 1
Switch Right	Reflux
Switch Left	Off
Switch Config1	Off
Switch Config2	Off

VIT 2
Switch Right	Reflux
Switch Left	Off
Switch Config1	Off
Switch Config2	Off

DIA
Switch Right	Off
Switch Left	Off
Switch Config1	Off
Switch Config2	Off

Thresholds
Center	5%, 30%, 60%
Feedback	YES
Sounds	Settings
Vacuum	6
Diathermy	6
Phaco Power	0
Error	6
Irrigation	3
Key Press	6
Speech	6
High Vacuum Sound	On
Mode Change	Voice
Submode Change	Voice
Value Change	On
Activity Confirmation	On

REFERENCES

1. Yao K, Tang XJ, Huang XD, Ye PP. Clinical evaluation on the bimanual microincision cataract surgery. *Zhonghua Yan Ke Za Zhi.* 2008;44(6):525-528.
2. Saeed A, O'Connor J, Cunnife G, Stack J, Mullhern MG, Beatty S. Uncorrected visual acuity in the immediate postoperative period following uncomplicated cataract surgery: bimanual microincision cataract surgery versus standard coaxial phacoemulsification. *Int Ophthalmol.* 2009;29(5):393-400.
3. Soscia W, Howard JG, Olson RJ. Microphacoemulsification with WhiteStar: a wound-temperature study. *J Cataract Refract Surg.* 2002;28(6):1044-1046.
4. Steinert RF, Schafer ME. Thermal energy and turbulence with Whitestar and conventional phacoemulsification. Paper presented at: ASCRS Annual Meeting: San Francisco, CA; April 12-16, 2003.
5. Soscia W, Howard JG, Olson RJ. Bimanual phacoemulsification through 2 stab incisions: a wound-temperature study. *J Cataract Refract Surg.* 2002;28(6):1039-1043.
6. Jiang Y, Liu Y, Cao Q. An experimental wound-temperature study of bimanual microphacoemulsification using the WhiteStar system. *Yan Ke Xue Bao.* 2005;21(2):122-125.
7. Donnenfeld ED, Olson RJ, Solomon R, et al. Efficacy and wound-temperature gradient of WhiteStar phacoemulsification through a 1.2 mm incision. *J Cataract Refract Surg.* 2003;29(6):1097-1100.
8. Olson RJ, Jin Y, Kefalopoulos G, Brinton J. Legacy AdvanTec and Sovereign WhiteStar: a wound temperature study. *J Cataract Refract Surg.* 2004;30(5):1109-1113.
9. Liu Y, Jiang Y, Wu M, Liu Y, Zhang T. Bimanual microincision phacoemulsification in treating hard cataracts using different power modes. *Clin Experiment Ophthalmol.* 2008;36(5):426-430.
10. Data on file, Abbott Medical Optics.
11. Assaf A, El-Matassem Kotb AM. Feasibility of bimanual microincision phacoemulsification in hard cataracts. *Eye.* 2007;21(6):807-811.
12. Olson RJ. Clinical experience with 21-gauge manual microphacoemulsification using Sovereign WhiteStar technology in eyes with dense cataract. *J Cataract Refract Surg.* 2004;30(1):168-172.
13. Vasavada AR, Mamidipudi PR, Minj M. Relationship of immediate intraocular pressure rise to phaco-tip ergonomics and energy dissipation. *J Cataract Refract Surg.* 2004;30(1):137-143.
14. Yoshida M. Ultra high speed images of phaco tip. Video presented at: ASCRS Annual Meeting: San Francisco, CA; March 17-22, 2006.
15. Fishkind W, Bakewell B, Donnenfeld ED, Rose AD, Watkins LA, Olson RJ. Comparative clinical trial of ultrasound phacoemulsification with and without the WhiteStar system. *J Cataract Refract Surg.* 2006;32(1):45-49.
16. Dewey, S. Increased control and efficiency; the next evolution of micropulse phaco. Paper presented at: ASCRS Annual Meeting: San Francisco, CA; March 17-22, 2006.
17. Georgescu D, Payne M, Olson RJ. Objective measurement of postocclusion surge during phacoemulsification in human eye bank eyes. *Am J Ophthalmol.* 2007;143(3):437-440.
18. Georgescu D, Kuo AF, Kinard KI, Olson RJ. A fluidics comparison of Alcon Infiniti, Bausch & Lomb Stellaris, and Advanced Medical Optics Signature phacoemulsification machines. *Am J Ophthalmol.* 2008;145(6):1014-1017.
19. Karaguzel H, Karalezli A, Aslan BS. Comparison of peristaltic and venturi pumps in bimanual microincisional cataract surgery. *Int Ophthalmol.* 2008, October 14.
20. Letter to editor. *Ophthalmol Times.* June 15, 2002.

SECTION III
MICS—SURGICAL TECHNIQUES

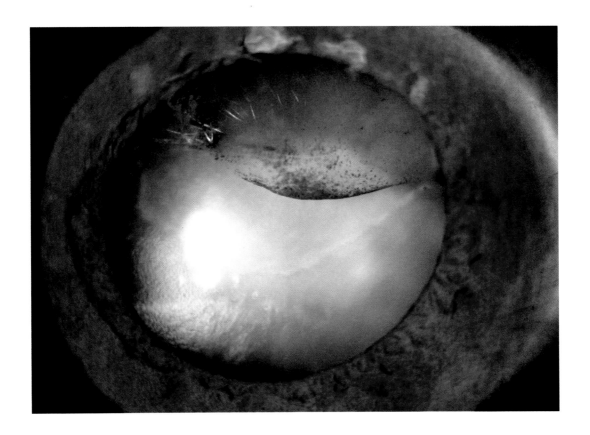

CHAPTER 8

Transition to Microincisional Cataract Surgery

Uday Devgan, MD, FACS, FRCS(Glasg)

With the move to smaller incisions, we need to adapt our surgical techniques to efficiently perform phacoemulsification.[1-7] Though the principles of surgery are the same in large- or small-incision phaco surgery, there are some key differences in instrumentation, fluidics, and lens insertion. Most experienced surgeons will be able to transition to microincisional cataract surgery (MICS) with a mild to moderate learning curve spanning just a few dozen cases.

INSTRUMENTATION

CORNEAL INCISIONS

With small incisions, we need to transition to smaller instruments, starting with smaller-gauge diamond or steel blades to create our incisions. For clear corneal incisions, the technique of making a square incision, where the tunnel length is approximately equal to the width of the incision, allows for better sealing of the wound. This is actually facilitated in MICS because the incision width is dramatically lessened.

Until a surgeon determines his ideal incision width, it is recommended to start with disposable steel keratomes because they are far less expensive than diamond blades. The technique of making the clear corneal incision is the same as with larger-gauge phacoemulsification, with single- and dual-plane configurations among the more common types. An incision that is too narrow will cause oar-locking and difficulty moving within the incision. An incision that is too wide will cause excessive leakage, which can lead to excessive fluid outflow and chamber instability and increases the risk for complications such as posterior capsule rupture (Figure 8-1).

CAPSULORRHEXIS

The capsulorrhexis forceps need to be placed through the smaller phaco incision, and this is a principle area of difference where the traditional cataract instruments need to be updated. Utrata-type capsulorrhexis forceps are typically too large for incisions of 2 mm or less. Some companies have developed Utrata forceps with ultrafine arms that will go through these smaller incisions. Alternatively, there are 25-gauge retina-style instruments that will even go through a 1-mm incision.

Agarwal A, Lindstrom R.
Microincisional Cataract Surgery: The Art and Science (pp 89-94).
© 2010 SLACK Incorporated

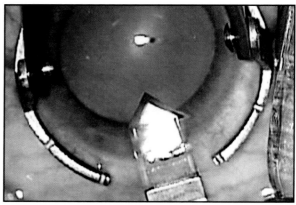

Figure 8-1. A diamond blade is used to create a square incision in the temporal cornea in preparation for phacoemulsification surgery.

In larger-incision surgery, the capsulorrhexis could be performed with mostly wrist movements. In contrast, with MICS, it is primarily fingertip movements. With these smaller-gauge instruments, it also becomes possible to perform the capsulorrhexis via the main incision or via the side-port paracentesis incision. This ability to switch hands can facilitate capsulorrhexis creation in challenging situations (Figure 8-2).

Phaco Needles and Sleeves

There is a range of phaco needle sizes that are used in MICS, ranging from 0.7 mm (also called 700 µm) to 1.1 mm. For a bimanual approach, these phaco needles are placed bare into the incision while the other hand uses an infusion device. For coaxial MICS, there is a need for a silicone phaco sleeve to allow for infusion via the same incision as aspiration.

Newer phaco sleeves are thinner and allow for sufficient levels of fluid flow into the eye. These are often color-coded by the manufacturers to aid in selection for surgery. During irrigation and aspiration of the lens cortex, the same principles apply and a bimanual approach may allow better access to the entire 360 degrees of the capsular bag. It is important to properly match the phaco needle, the infusion sleeve, and the incision size in order to achieve fluidic balance, safety, and efficiency during surgery.

Adjusting the Phaco Fluidics

Due to the small volume of the anterior and posterior chambers, the control of fluidics during phacoemulsification surgery is important to ensure efficient removal of the cataract while preventing complications due to tissue collapse. With microincisional surgery, the primary challenge is keeping the inflow of fluid sufficiently higher.

The basic concept of fluidics is that the inflow of fluid must be greater than the outflow of fluid. By keeping a constant infusion pressure and limiting the outflow, we can ensure that the eye stays inflated and stable during surgery. If we allow the outflow to exceed the fluid inflow, even for just a fraction of a second, we experience surge within the eye and this can cause chamber instability, collapse of the eye, and aspiration of the posterior capsule. The primary rule for phaco fluidics is to keep the inflow greater than the outflow.

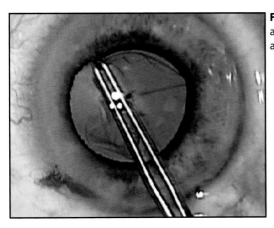

Figure 8-2. Capsulorrhexis forceps with thinner arms are able to be used through a 2-mm incision without a problem.

Modulating Phaco Fluid Flow: Poiseuille's Equation

The basic equation that governs all fluid flow during phacoemulsification surgery is Poiseuille's equation:

$$F = \Delta P \pi r^4 / 8 \eta L$$

In this equation, F = flow, ΔP = pressure gradient, r = radius of the tube, η = viscosity of fluid, and L = length of the tube. We are concerned with the relative relationship and not the exact values; therefore, for simplicity, we can simplify this formula. The viscosity of the fluid is relatively constant, as is the length of the tubing. The values of pi and 8 are constant. This leaves us with a simpler equation:

$$F \sim \Delta P r^4$$

Flow is proportional to the change in pressure times the radius of the tubing to the fourth power. Because the value for tubing size is exponential, a small change to the radius results in a large change in the relative flow.

Modulating Fluid Inflow

The source of fluid inflow is the bottle of balanced salt solution that is hanging on the phaco machine. The 2 factors that determine the rate of inflow are the change in pressure and the radius of the inflow tubing. The change in pressure can be modulated by raising or lowering the height of the bottle relative to the patient's eye: the higher the bottle, the higher the infusion pressure. The inflow tubing has a large radius in order to maximize the flow and make sure that we keep our inflow greater than the outflow. Similarly, the size of the infusion channel within the phaco probe (or other infusion instrument) is kept as large as possible in order to avoid a bottleneck effect.

Modulating Fluid Outflow

For fluid outflow, there are 2 sources of fluid leaving the eye: (1) the fluid that is removed via the phaco probe as a result of the vacuum level generated by the fluid pump and (2) fluid leakage from the incisions.

The rate of the fluid outflow via the phaco needle is determined by the radius of the needle and tubing, as well as the change in pressure generated by the phaco machine's fluid pump. The rate of the fluid outflow loss via the incisions depends on their size and the relative fit of the instruments within these incisions.

Some degree of fluid leakage from the incisions is helpful to allow cooling of the phaco needle and to prevent thermal injury during surgery, particularly early in the learning stages of phacoemulsification. With the use of advanced phaco power modulations, more experienced phaco surgeons tend to move toward tighter incisions, which can give more stable fluidics.

Surge is the situation when the outflow of fluid from the eye exceeds the inflow, even for just a fraction of a second. When this occurs, the chamber tends to collapse and the posterior capsule can be sucked into the phaco probe in an instant, resulting in a ruptured posterior capsule and vitreous loss.

In order to maintain this flow balance, where the inflow is always greater than the outflow, we can use different sized tubing. If we look at the inflow tubing, we notice that it is significantly different than the outflow tubing.

PHACO NEEDLE SIZING

The size of the phaco needle is important for phaco fluidics because it affects the outflow rate. The important thing to remember from Poiseuille's equation is that the flow is proportional to the radius of the tube to the fourth power. This means that a small change in the size of the phaco needle can result in a very large change in the flow. Comparing 2 common-sized phaco needles, 0.9 mm versus 1.1 mm, with all other factors equal, it is surprising to see that the flow through the larger 1.1-mm needle is more than twice that of the 0.9-mm needle. As the needle size decreases, the flow drops exponentially.

If we switch from a 1.1-mm phaco needle to a 0.9-mm needle, with all other phaco parameters unchanged, the relative flow will decrease by more than half to 45% of the relative flow through the 1.1-mm needle. In order to achieve the same flow while decreasing the needle size, a substantial increase in the pressure gradient is required. This can be achieved by raising the bottle height and using gravity as the infusion force or, alternatively, a forced infusion can be created by using a pump to push fluid into the eye or pressurizing the bottle using an air pump.

Once we determine the proper tubing size and phaco needle size for our needs, we can then select the other parameters of the phaco machine. Remember that the tubing size and phaco needle size are definitely variables that play an important role in the fluidics.

INTRAOCULAR LENS INSERTION

Once the cataract has been fully removed and the capsular bag is empty, it is time for intraocular lens (IOL) insertion. This can be accomplished by inserting the IOL through the existing microincision, enlarging the incision, or creating a new incision.

For IOL insertion using the existing microincision, there are multiple choices described elsewhere in this book. The concept of wound-assist places the IOL injector tip up against the corneal incision but not inside it. The corneal tunnel then acts as an extension of the injector tip and the IOL can be passed through the cornea and into the eye. This allows the IOL to go through a smaller incision because the added bulk of the injector tip is not placed inside the corneal incision. Care must be taken, however, to avoid exposure of the IOL to the tear film because this may introduce bacteria into the anterior chamber at the conclusion of the case (Figure 8-3).

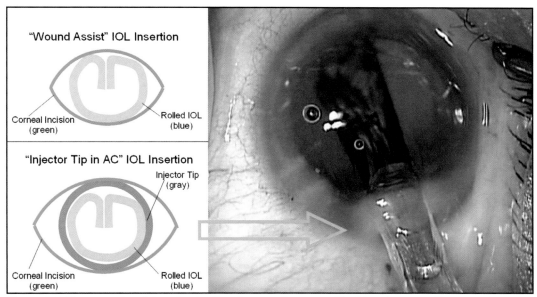

Figure 8-3. The wound-assist methods allow for a smaller corneal incision; however, there may be exposure to tear film contaminants. By placing the injector tip into the anterior chamber, the single-piece acrylic intraocular lens is injected into the capsular bag. Using this slightly larger incision allows for a smooth, controlled delivery while keeping the intraocular lens away from the tear film and associated contaminants.

The incision can be enlarged to allow a more comfortable delivery of the IOL into the eye. This may increase the astigmatic effect of the incision, so care should be taken to widen the incision only as much as required. Finally, an entirely new incision can be created for IOL insertion. This is sometimes done with bimanual MICS such as 700-μm cataract surgery described by Agarwal.

The move toward smaller incisions has benefited both patients and surgeons, and we are currently at the sweet spot, where the incisions are large enough for controlled, efficient surgery and IOL insertion but small enough to seal well and produce minimal astigmatic effects. When evaluating your own patients and surgical results, make sure that the incisions seal well and have a predictable astigmatic effect.

SUMMARY

The transition to MICS is an important step for the cataract surgeon to evolve his technique. The move is toward less invasive and safer, more predictable surgery. With a little bit of careful planning and a few modifications to our instruments, fluidic settings, and lens insertion techniques, it is a transition that all cataract surgeons can make.

REFERENCES

1. Agarwal A, Agarwal A, Agarwal S, Narang P, Narang S. Phakonit: phacoemulsification through a 0.9 mm corneal incision. *J Cataract Refract Surg.* 2001;27(10):1548-1552.
2. Fine IH, Hoffman RS, Packer M. Profile of clear corneal cataract incisions demonstrated by ocular coherence tomography. *J Cataract Refract Surg.* 2007;33(1):94-97.
3. May W, Castro-Combs J, Camacho W, Wittmann P, Behrens A. Analysis of clear corneal incision integrity in an ex vivo model. *J Cataract Refract Surg.* 2008;34(6):1013-1018.

CHAPTER 8

4. Poiseuille JLM. Recherches expérimentales sur le mouvement de liquides dans les tubes de très petits diamètres. *Mémoires présentés par divers savants à l'Académie des Sciences Paris.* 1846;9:433-543.
5. Sutera SP, Skalak R. The history of Poiseuille's Law. *Annu Rev Fluid Mech.* 1993;25:1-20.
6. Koch P. *Mastering Phacoemulsification: A Simplified Manual of Strategies for the Spring, Crack and Stop and Chop Technique.* 4th Ed. Thorofare, NJ: SLACK Incorporated; 1993.
7. Kelman CD. Phaco-emulsification and aspiration: A new technique of cataract removal: A preliminary report. *Am J Ophthalmol.* 1967;64(1):23-35.

CHAPTER 9

MICROCOAXIAL PHACOEMULSIFICATION

*Vaishali Vasavada, MS; Viraj A. Vasavada, MS;
Abhay R. Vasavada, MS, FRCS; and Shetal M. Raj, DO, MS*

Modern cataract surgery has undergone a series of remarkable technical refinements. Many of these advances have focused on technologies that involve a change in the type and size of the incision. Small incisions are associated with faster patient rehabilitation, improved prognosis for visual acuity, and reduced surgically induced astigmatism.[1,2] These smaller incisions also increase wound stability, reduce ocular trauma, and reduce the risk of iris prolapse. Currently, there are 2 popular small-incision phacoemulsification techniques: bimanual phacoemulsification and coaxial microincisional cataract surgery (C-MICS; microcoaxial phacoemulsification).

BIMANUAL MICROINCISIONAL CATARACT SURGERY

Bimanual microincisional cataract surgery (B-MICS) requires 2 incisions, each smaller than 1.5 mm, in order to perform emulsification. In this technique started by Amar Agarwal, the irrigation and aspiration are separated from each other,[3-5] and 2 paracentesis incisions ranging from 1.2 to 1.5 mm are made to accommodate the sleeveless phacoemulsificaiton tip and the irrigating chopper. This technique was introduced with the purpose of reducing the incision size; however, one of the major limitations of this technique is that the surgeon often has to enlarge the incision[5-7] or create a third incision[8,9] in order to implant an intraocular lens (IOL) of 6.0-mm optic. Alternatively, the surgeon would have to use an IOL that can be implanted without enlarging the incison.[10,11] IOLs designed for implantation through the MICS incision are still evolving and do not have a proven track record. The use of multifocal IOLS, aspherical IOLs, and spherical IOLs with proven optic and edge designs and materials through microincisions in the bimanual technique still remains an issue.[5]

CONVENTIONAL COAXIAL PHACOEMULSIFICATION

Conventional coaxial phacoemulsification requires a 2.8- to 3.5-mm–wide incision to insert a phaco tip with a silicone sleeve through a single valvular incision for coaxial aspiration and irrigation.[12,13] This silicone sleeve acts to cool the tip, and it seals and protects the incision from thermal injury when performing phacoemulsification.

Microincisional Coaxial Phacoemulsification

A recent development in coaxial phacoemulsification facilitates IOL implantation through a 2.2-mm incision. This technique, which is referred to as microcoaxial phacoemulsification or C-MICS, requires an incision of 2.2 mm or less and accommodates a sleeved phaco tip. This allows aspiration and irrigation through the same incision coaxially and allows implantation of a full-sized IOL without enlarging the incision. This technique offers all of the advantages of standard coaxial surgery with the added benefit of using a small incision. From a clinical perspective, C-MICS involves a minimal learning curve and it provides favorable fluidics, a stable anterior chamber, and excellent postoperative outcomes.[14,15]

The Microcoaxial Incision

One of the most critical steps in contemporary cataract surgery is the creation of a clear corneal incision. Even with the adoption of small-incision cataract extraction techniques, wound integrity is a concern. There have been reports of increased incidence of endophthalmitis following inception of clear corneal incisions.[16] It has been suggested that poorly constructed and distorted wounds may increase the risk of postoperative endophthalmitis. Although smaller wounds would self-seal more easily, this is possible only if wound morphology and integrity are maintained. Small-incision phacoemulsification techniques often use tight wound geometry, which may give rise to "oar locking" and lead to difficulties in intraocular manipulations. At times, such geometry adds stress to the incision, leading to wound distortion, corneal hydration, and thermal injury.

It has been suggested that with phacoemulsification techniques employing clear corneal incisions, construction and integrity of the incision at the end of the surgery play a pivotal role in the reported increased rates of infection. It is therefore crucial to have a square or nearly square architecture of the incision and employ a surgical technique that minimizes incision distortion. Our previous randomized experimental study of rabbits' eyes found that, immediately after surgery, incisions used for sleeveless phacoemulsification had greater collagen damage on histomorphological and immunohistochemical analysis than the incisions used for sleeved-tip phacoemulsification.[17] In another clinical study, we found that ingress of trypan blue from the ocular surface into the anterior chamber was found to be less with microincisional coaxial incisions compared to bimanual phacoemulsification.[18]

With C-MICS, a single-plane, temporal, clear corneal incision of 2.0 to 2.2 mm is created using a sharp trapezoidal keratome placed parallel to the dome of the cornea, making the internal entry in a single motion. It is of utmost importance to pay attention to the architecture and design of the incision. For a microcoaxial incision of 2.2-mm width, an internal entry of at least 1.5 mm is mandatory to ensure good self-sealing nature of the wound (Figure 9-1). More importantly, there should be minimal stress and distortion of the incision during intraocular manipulations.

Surgical Technique and Instrumentation

Surgery is performed using a conventional 0.9-mm phaco tip with specially modified smaller diameter sleeves—the Ultra Sleeve and the Nanosleeve (Alcon, Fort Worth, TX). With C-MICS (Figure 9-2), there is a reduction in fluid inflow into the eye by about 30%. This reduced inflow, in turn, restricts the limit to which the aspiration flow rate can be increased. The lower irrigation flow is compensated for by thinner sleeve designs as well

MICROCOAXIAL PHACOEMULSIFICATION

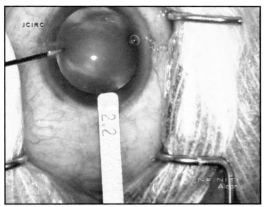

Figure 9-1. Single-plane clear corneal incision measuring 2.2 mm.

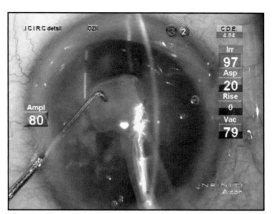

Figure 9-2. Microincisional coaxial phacoemulsification.

as innovations in ultrasound modulations, innovative phaco tip designs, raising the bottle height, and improved tubing/cassettes with superior fluid dynamics.

One of the merits of this technique is that surgeons can use their conventional instruments and techniques. It is not necessary to have expensive side-port capsulorrhexis forceps or to use unfamiliar irrigating choppers. The technique of nucleus emulsification remains the same as in coaxial phacoemulsification. Our technique of choice is the step-by-step chop in situ and lateral separation[19] technique, because it allows division of nuclear fragments within the area of the capsulorrhexis, with minimal stress to the zonules. Whatever the technique of nucleus division, fragment removal should be confined to a posterior plane as far as possible (Figure 9-3), thereby minimizing damage to the corneal endothelium. Further, using lower fluidic parameters and progressively reducing them by adhering to the principles of slow motion technique[20] and step-down technique[21] allows the surgeon to perform fragment removal safely at the posterior plane (Figure 9-4).

INTRAOCULAR LENS IMPLANTATION

IOL implantation can be performed using a plunger-type injection system and the appropriate cartridge with the wound-assisted injection technique (Figure 9-5). Even though the cartridge does not pass through the internal entry of the 2.0/2.2-mm incision, it suffices to place the cartridge at the outer edge of the incision and use the plunger to implant the lens into the eye. The key point is to provide counterforce to the cartridge. Keeping a rigid ocular tension during implantation is another important point. Typically, there is an enlargement by about 1 mm following implantation of the IOL (Figure 9-6). Newer cartridges (eg, Monarch D cartridge, Alcon) allow IOL implantation through these incisions (Figure 9-7).

POWER MODULATIONS

With the advent of ultrasound power modulations, performing C-MICS has become safer and more efficient. Several modulations of traditional ultrasound are now available, such as the pulse mode, burst mode, hyperpulse mode, WhiteStar technology (Abbott Medical Optics, Santa Ana, CA), WhiteStar ICE technology, and others. All of these modulations allow interrupted use of ultrasound energy, thus minimizing heat-induced damage to these small incisions, as well as making emulsification more efficient.

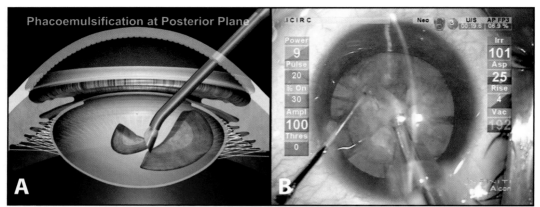

Figures 9-3. (A) Schematic representation of nuclear fragment removal within the capsular bag. (B) Fragment removal being performed at posterior plane, away from the corneal endothelium.

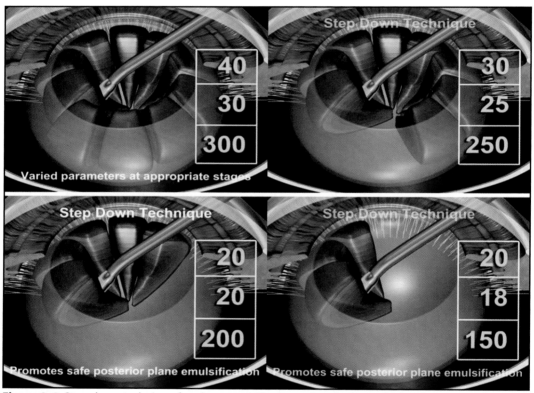

Figure 9-4. Step-down technique for phacoemulsification, wherein the aspiration flow rate and vacuum are progressively reduced as the posterior capsule is exposed.

Newer ultrasound delivery modalities have come up, such as torsional ultrasound (OZil, Alcon) and transverse ultrasound (Ellipse, Abbott Medical Optics), which allow ultrasound energy to be used much more efficiently. The torsional ultrasound (OZil) involves transverse oscillations of the phaco tip at a frequency of 32 000 Hz. This results in excellent followability with minimal repulsion of lens material, thereby allowing more efficient and faster emulsification. Combination torsional ultrasound with C-MICS is extremely beneficial, particularly in dense cataracts and other difficult scenarios.

MICROCOAXIAL PHACOEMULSIFICATION

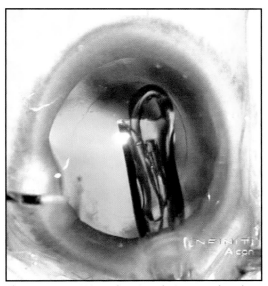

Figure 9-5. Wound-assisted intraocular lens implantation with the cartridge placed halfway in the corneal tunnel. Counterforce is provided by the second instrument.

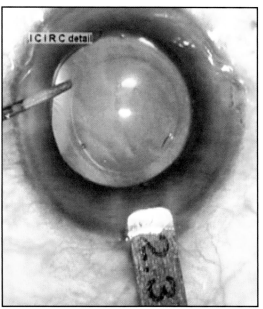

Figure 9-6. Incision enlargement by 0.1 mm following intraocular lens implantation.

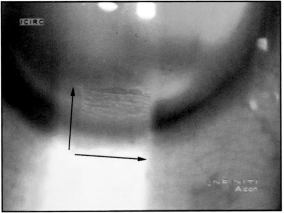

Figure 9-7. Microcoaxial phaco incision.

COAXIAL MICROINCISIONAL CATARACT SURGERY IN DIFFICULT SITUATIONS

C-MICS (Figure 9-8) can be performed to emulsify cataracts in eyes with a compromised endothelium, small pupil, and weak zonules, as well as those with posterior polar cataracts, subluxated cataracts, and other difficult cataracts.

DENSE CATARACT AND COAXIAL MICROINCISIONAL CATARACT SURGERY

Major concerns in dense cataract emulsification are corneal endothelial damage and wound site thermal injury due to excessive dissipation of ultrasound energy, especially with smaller incisions. With C-MICS, there is some reduction in irrigation, and we need to have lower fluidic parameters to be more effective in order to perform posterior plane emulsification. C-MICS, in combination with torsional ultrasound, is a boon for dense

Figure 9-8. Sleeves used in microcoaxial phaco.

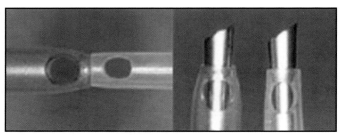

cataract emulsification; energy and aspiration work in harmony with OZil and microcoaxial because there is minimal to no repulsion of the lens substance—it stays at the tip. Using the Kelman tip (Alcon) with 45-degree bevel with torsional phaco through a 2.1- or 2.2-mm incision is the best combination to tackle dense cataracts. What is more striking is that the incision at the end of phaco is undistorted, and there is no incisional hydration or stress seen. This will ensure clearer corneas on postoperative day 1 consistently.

MIOTIC PUPIL

A small pupil affects all steps of phacoemulsification, from capsulorrhexis to IOL insertion. Difficult maneuvering causes iris damage, sphincter tears, zonular dialysis, bleeding, and so on. Poor exposure through a small pupil forces the surgeon to make a smaller rhexis, adding further to the difficulty and frequently leading to capsular dehiscence and nucleus drop—the worst nightmare. The prolonged surgical time takes its toll thereafter (corneal edema, uveitis, secondary glaucoma, cystoid macular edema, distorted pupil—the list is endless). All of these lead to poor visual outcome, an unhappy patient, and a frustrated surgeon.

PREOPERATIVE

A good surgeon should not wait unprepared to deal with the devil on the operating table.

A preoperative evaluation should include pupillary dynamics. Poor pupillary dilatation should be detected and noted. Appropriate history is important for detecting any underlying etiology for the miotic pupil, whether it is the use of miotics or long-standing diabetes. Any coexisting conditions like zonular weakness in pseudo-exfoliation or synechiae in chronic uveitis should be detected preoperatively. The pupil should be dilated with a combination of cycloplegic, mydriatic, and nonsteroidal anti-inflammatory drops.

SPHINCTER SPARING TECHNIQUES

Pharmacological mydriasis alone may not be effective in cases with posterior synechiae, pupillary membrane, or scarred pupils. Such pupils need intraoperative procedures. High-molecular-weight cohesive viscoelastics such as sodium hyaluronate (Healon-5 or Healon GV) can be injected into the center of the pupil to mechanically dissect any synechiae and to stretch the sphincter. If this does not work, synechiolysis may be done with a blunt spatula passed through the side-port incision. Viscomydriasis can then be repeated. Pupillary membranes can be stripped mechanically by the Utrata forceps. Pure, preservative-free adrenaline can be added to the irrigation bottle after appropriate dilatation. Care should be taken in hypertensives and the irrigating solution should be immediately changed to an adrenaline-free solution in case of a posterior capsular rupture.

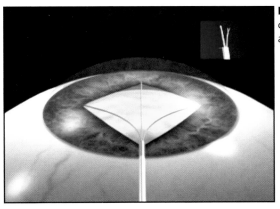

Figure 9-9. Tripronged pupil stretchers. (Photo courtesy of Dr. Agarwal's Group of Eye Hospitals and Eye Research Centre, Chennai, India.)

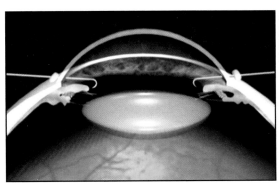

Figure 9-10. Iris hooks inserted to enlarge the pupil. (Photo courtesy of Dr. Agarwal's Group of Eye Hospitals and Eye Research Centre, Chennai, India.)

SPHINCTER INVOLVING TECHNIQUES

Mini sphincterotomies, less than 1 mm, and limited to the sphincter tissue can be made with either Vannas scissors (Appasamy Associates, Chennai, India) or the vitreoretinal scissors. This gives adequate dilatation intraoperatively and maintains a functionally and esthetically normal pupil postoperatively. The disadvantage is that the incision is more difficult to create in the clock hour of the wound.

Dilatation can also be achieved by pupillary stretching using push–pull instruments. Under viscoelastic cover, 2 hooks are used in a slow, simultaneous, and controlled fashion to stretch the pupil in one or more axes. Bipronged, tripronged, and quadripronged pupil stretchers are also effective (Figure 9-9). The prongs should be maintained parallel to the iris plane and should not slip out into the pupil margin, especially on starting to depress the plunger to create the pupil stretch. The disadvantage of pupil stretch techniques is that the iris sometimes becomes flaccid and prolapses through the incision during surgery. Postoperatively, the pupil usually remains esthetically acceptable.

In very small pupils, commercially available iris hooks can be used to stretch the pupil (Figure 9-10). Gradual and optimal enlargement of the pupil to a size just adequate for the surgery should be attempted to avoid pupillary atony. The hooks should be placed parallel to the iris plane through small, short, peripheral paracentesis. If not placed properly, they can pull the iris diaphragm forward, resulting in chafing and thermal damage during phacoemulsification of the nucleus.

The Malyugin ring (MicroSurgical Technology, Redmond, WA) is another great device to help surgery in small pupils (Figure 9-11).

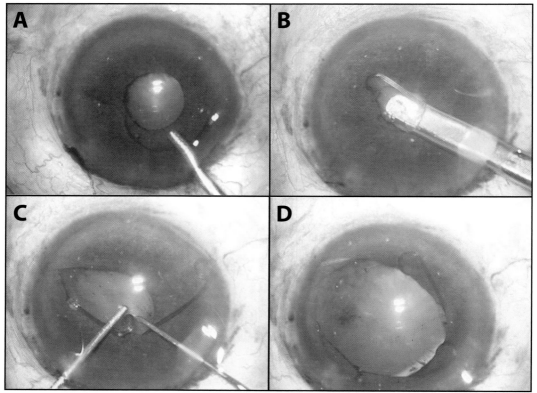

Figures 9-11. Steps of Malyugin ring for small-pupil phaco surgery. (Photo courtesy of Dr. Agarwal's Group of Eye Hospitals and Eye Research Centre, Chennai, India.)

Summary

This new era of microcoaxial surgery will enhance patient outcomes by minimizing surgically induced astigmatism, theoretically provide a potent barrier against postoperative infection, and encourage faster postoperative visual recovery.

References

1. Linebarger EJ, Hardten DR, Shah GK, Lindstrom RL. Phacoemulsification and modern cataract surgery. *Surv Ophthalmol.* 1999;44(2):123-147.
2. Dick HB, Schwenn C, Krummenauer F, Krist R, Pfeiffer N. Inflammation after sclerocorneal versus clear corneal tunnel phacoemulsification. *Ophthalmology.* 2000;107(2):241-247.
3. Tsuneoka H, Shiba T, Takahashi Y. Feasibility of ultrasound cataract surgery with a 1.4 mm incision. *J Cataract Refract Surg.* 2001;27(6):934-940.
4. Agarwal A, Agarwal S, Agarwal A, Narang P, Narang S. Phakonit: phacoemulsification through a 0.9 mm corneal incision. *J Cataract Refract Surg.* 2001;27(10):1548-1552.
5. Tsuneoka H, Shiba T, Takahashi Y. Ultrasonic phacoemulsification using a 1.4 mm incision: clinical results. *J Cataract Refract Surg.* 2002;28(1):81-86.
6. Donnenfeld ED, Olson RJ, Solomon R, et al. Efficacy and wound-temperature gradient of WhiteStar phacoemulsification through a 1.2 mm incision. *J Cataract Refract Surg.* 2003;29(6):1097-1100.
7. Tsuneoka H, Hayama A, Takahama M. Ultrasmall-incision bimanual phacoemulsification and Acrysof SA30AL implantation through a 2.2 mm incision. *J Cataract Refract Surg.* 2003;29(6):1070-1076.
8. Fine IH, Hoffman RS, Packer M. Optimizing refractive lens exchange with bimanual microincision phacoemulsification. *J Cataract Refract Surg.* 2004;30(3):550-554.

9. Assaf A, El-Moatassem Kotb AM. Feasibility of bimanual micro-incision phacoemulsification in hard cataracts. *Eye*. 2007;21(6):807-811.
10. Alió JL, Rodríguez-Prats JL, Galal A, Ramzy M. Outcomes of microincision cataract surgery versus coaxial phacoemulsification. *Ophthalmology*. 2005;112(11):1997-2003.
11. Alió JL, Rodríguez-Prats J-L, Vianello A, Galal A. Visual outcome of microincision cataract surgery with implantation of an Acri.Smart lens. *J Cataract Refract Surg*. 2005;31:1549-1556.
12. Dholakia SA, Vasavada AR. Intraoperative performance and longterm outcome of phacoemulsification in age-related cataract. *Indian J Ophthalmol*. 2004;52:311-317.
13. Dholakia SA, Vasavada AR, Singh R. Prospective evaluation of phacoemulsification in adults younger than 50 years. *J Cataract Refract Surg*. 2005;31(7):1327-1333.
14. Vasavada V, Vasavada V, Raj SM, Vasavada AR. Intraoperative performance and postoperative outcomes of microcoaxial phacoemulsification: observational study. *J Cataract Refract Surg*. 2007;33(6):1019-1024.
15. Osher RH. Microcoaxial phacoemulsificaiton part 2: clinical study. *J Cataract Refract Surg*. 2007;33(3):408-412.
16. Taban M, Behrens A, Newcomb RL, et al. Acute endophthalmitis following cataract surgery: a systematic review of the literature. *Arch Ophthalmol*. 2005;123(5):613-620.
17. Johar SR, Vasavada AR, Praveen MR, et al. Histomorphological and immunofluorescence evaluation of bimanual and coaxial phacoemulsification in rabbits. *J Cataract Refract Surg*. 2008;34(4):670-676.
18. Praveen MR, Vasavada AR, Gajjar D, et al. Comparative quantification of ingress of trypan blue into the anterior chamber after microcoaxial, standard coaxial, and bimanual phacoemulsification: randomized clinical trial. *J Cataract Refract Surg*. 2008;34(6):1007-1012.
19. Vasavada A, Singh R. Step-by-step chop in situ and separation of very dense cataracts. *J Cataract Refract Surg*. 1998:24(2):156-159.
20. Osher RH. Slow motion phacoemulsification approach. *J Cataract Refract Surg*. 1993;19(5):667.
21. Vasavada AR, Raj S. Step-down technique. *J Cataract Refract Surg*. 2003;29(6):1077-1079.

CHAPTER 10

Sub-2-mm Lens Surgery

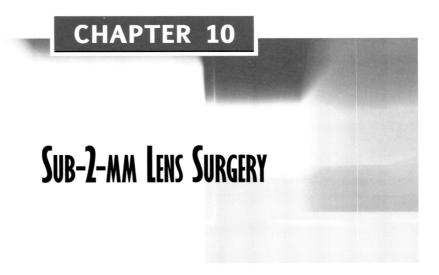

Richard Packard, MD, DO, FRCS, FRCOphth

When Harold Ridley first implanted a lens in 1949, the incision size for cataract surgery was about 12 mm. This was the norm until Charles Kelman introduced phacoemulsification in the late 1960s, when it became possible to remove a cataract through a wound of 3.5 mm. The lenses available at the time were very limited, however, and required enlarging the incision to at least 7 mm. In 1985, Tom Mazzocco pioneered the first foldable lens—the STAAR AA4003 (Monrovia, CA) with plate haptics—which was able to go through that 3.5-mm incision. The original lens had a number of drawbacks and was slow to be adopted. In 1988, the first foldable lens approved by the US Food and Drug Administration was the SI18 made by Abbott Medical Optics (Santa Ana, CA). During the late 1980s and early 1990s, any number of new foldable designs appeared, most notably the AcrySof (Alcon, Fort Worth, TX) series of hydrophobic intraocular lenses (IOLs). Although the incision size reduced to 3 mm and then 2.75 mm, the change was slow. It was limited by 3 major factors. Firstly, the phaco technology meant that power delivery and fluidics were not really up to anything smaller. More importantly, though, IOLs could not be delivered through smaller incisions.

Although Amar Agarwal introduced phakonit in 1998,[1-5] most surgeons were reluctant to move to bimanual surgery with separation of irrigation and aspiration for the phaco stage of the procedure. In Europe, bimanual irrigation and aspiration had already started to become popular by the late 1990s. It was the arrival of power modulation, in the form of very short pulses separated by variable intervals, first seen on the Allergan (now Abbott Medical Optics) Sovereign and called WhiteStar that changed our view of incision size. Suddenly it seemed safe to use a bare needle for phacoemulsification with separate irrigation via a separate incision using a specially designed chopper. IOLs quickly started to appear for these 1.5-mm incisions and microincisional cataract surgery (MICS) was born. The companies involved (ThinOptX, Abingdon, VA and Acri.Tec, Berlin, Germany) made lenses for these incisions but they were not to prove popular. This was partly because most surgeons were unwilling to acquire the tools and learn the new skills for operating through these very small incisions. The other issue was that the perceived benefit of moving from an incision of 2.75 to 3.00 mm to implant with what many felt might be an implant with inferior behavior was not apparent.

In 2005, Takyuki Akahoshi showed that coaxial phacoemulsification could be performed through a 2.2-mm incision with appropriate needles and sleeves. More importantly, he showed that using a wound-assisted technique, a standard 6-mm optic IOL could be implanted through this same unopened incision. Thus, micro-coaxial or coaxial MICS (C-MICS) was created. Due to the developments in machines, tips, sleeves, fluidics, lenses, and lens delivery systems, sub-2-mm C-MICS is now not only possible, but doable for any surgeon who understands the benefits of smaller incisions.

Reasons for Considering Sub-2-mm Coaxial Microincisional Cataract Surgery

Having demonstrated that it was possible to carry out cataract surgery through these smaller incisions, it became necessary to justify reasons other than the fact that we can. Many studies have shown little difference in ultimate outcome for the patient. Certain things stand out in favor of sub-2-mm surgery, of which lack of induced astigmatism and more rapid stabilization of the cornea are the most important. If correction for astigmatism, whether by toric lenses or using limbal relaxing incisions, is envisaged, it should be more predictable when incisions are smaller. From the patient's point of view, this means seeing better earlier and a stronger, less distortable wound.

The advocates of bimanual surgery are vociferous and eloquent in stating that separating irrigation from phaco and aspiration is the best way to perform nuclear removal. To date, however, there has been less-than-enthusiastic support from the majority of surgeons. The use of C-MICS, as envisaged by Akahoshi, seems to them to be a more attractive alternative to achieve smaller incisions. There is now technology available from a variety of companies that will allow safe and predictable sub-2-mm C-MICS.

Tools for Coaxial Microincisional Cataract Surgery

KNIVES

Side-Port Knife

Although many knives are available for the side port, this author prefers to use a 15-degree knife. The way that the blade is configured creates a trapezoidal incision that is ideal for the custom-designed disposable bimanual irrigation and aspiration currently preferred. The incision should be made at 2 o'clock, 60 degrees from the main wound, not as a stab but in a structured way by changing the hand position. It should also be over square from the limbus into the cornea. The incision is stopped as the end of the sharp part of the blade is reached to create the trapezoidal shape. This allows good movement of the instruments in the eye, with sealing only taking place at the internal ostium; thus, stretching is minimal.

The second side port is made at 9 o'clock if the surgeon is sitting at 12:00.

After the side-port incisions are made, the eye should be filled with viscoelastic to create a firm eye for the main wound. Although some prefer to use more viscous viscoelastics for routine cases, sodium hyaluronate 1% (Provisc, Healon, Biolon) is adequate. This will be discussed further later.

Slit Knife

As the phaco wound gets smaller, the knives needed to create that wound need to behave a little differently. Tissue resistance increases relatively with a smaller incision so that the angle of attack of the blade needs to be more acute. Further, many of the blades currently available provide resistance to passage through the tissues at the beginning of blade passage, which then suddenly is lost. This means that the surgeon loses control of the architecture of the wound. This author has designed a new blade specifically for 2.2- and 1.8-mm incisions to overcome these issues called the Windsor Knife (Core Surgical, Buckinghamshire, England). The blade is used in 4 hand positions to redirect it to create a 3-plane incision that rarely requires any hydration to seal (Figure 10-1). The ideal cross-sectional appearance for good sealing of an incision is seen in Figure 10-2.

VISCOELASTICS

As already mentioned, a relatively low-viscosity cohesive viscoelastic works well for most routine cases. The reason for using this is the ease of leakage during hydrodissection so that the eye does not become overpressurized and blow out the posterior capsule. If there is a hard cataract or the endothelium needs extra protection, a dispersive viscoelastic-like Viscoat (Alcon) can be used. It is important in this case to bleed some off before the hydrodissection. A cohesive viscoelastic like Provisc or Healon can be inserted after hydrodissection under the Viscoat to create the "soft shell" before the phacoemulsification begins. If Viscoat or any dispersive viscoelastic has been used without a soft shell, some must be removed from above the capsulorrhexis using aspiration before any ultrasound power is used. This avoids the possibility of an early occlusion, with ultrasound power in use, which can lead to a wound burn in just a few seconds.

CAPSULORRHEXIS

These very small incisions may mean that standard capsulorrhexis forceps will not work well because the blades cannot open enough. Using a needle is, of course, possible and there are a number of either coaxial micro-forceps or cross-action forceps (Calladine-Inamura Round Handle Capsulorrhexis Forceps, Duckworth & Kent, Hertfordshire, England) now available that will work well (Figure 10-3). The smaller incision will be helpful to retain viscoelastic in the eye during the capsulorrhexis.

HYDRODISSECTION

As already mentioned, it is important to avoid excess pressure in the eye during this step. Surgeons are advised to bleed off some viscoelastic prior to injecting balanced salt solution. This applies regardless of which cannula is used.

PHACO TIPS AND SLEEVES

Two companies, Bausch & Lomb (Aliso Viejo, CA) and Oertli (Berneck, Switzerland), have designed and are promoting sub-2-mm C-MICS. They have sleeves that allow the tip to work through small incisions that come with their tips for C-MICS (Bausch & Lomb Devine tip at 1.8 mm and Oertli Smart tip at 1.6 mm). As less fluid is able to enter the eye, a smaller tip is required to allow adequate irrigation for a stable anterior chamber. Both of these tips have narrower shafts than the entry point to the tip. The Bausch & Lomb tip has an internal diameter of 500 µm, whereas the Oertli tip is only 400 µm. Although this creates greater resistance to flow and thus less surge after occlusion break, speed of nuclear removal and clogging can be an issue.

Alcon has so far favored an incision size of 2.2 mm using the Ultra Sleeve. They have a sleeve for use at 1.8 mm called the Nano Sleeve that has not yet been released. This author has considerable experience with this. The tips available for this are the same as those for 2.2 mm and are all in some way curved to act with torsional phaco (OZil, Alcon). As well as being curved, all are flared with an internal diameter at the narrowest point of 570 µm.

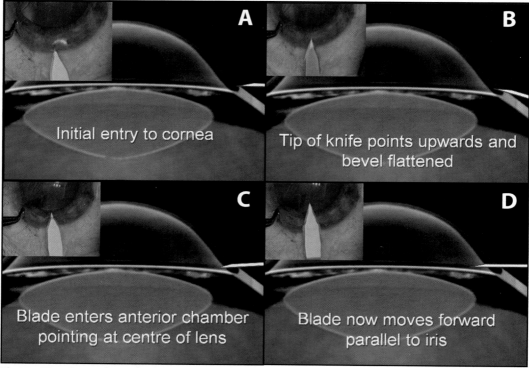

Figure 10-1. Steps of creating a clear corneal incision.

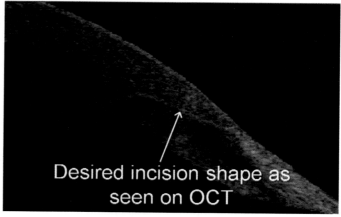

Figure 10-2. Clear corneal incision as seen on anterior segment optical coherence tomography.

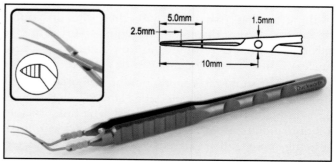

Figure 10-3. Cross-action capsulorrhexis forceps. (Reprinted with permission from Duckworth & Kent, Hertfordshire, England.)

In a number of studies, it has been shown that although all bevels of these mini-flared tips will work reasonably well for soft and medium cataracts, this is not true of denser nuclei. Only the 45-degree mini-flared tip seemed to be almost immune to clogging during segment removal. The recent upgrade for the Infiniti phaco machine with Intelligent Phaco software, which allows a short burst of longitudinal power to clear unwanted occlusions, has enabled the 30-degree Miniflared tip to deal with hard nuclei more efficiently. The problem with both the 45 degree tip and the tip on the Oertli machine, which has a bevel of 53 degrees, is difficulty in chopping and obtaining occlusion for segment removal. For those surgeons who use a 4-quadrant nucleofractis technique, this is not an issue.

PACKARD 700-µM KELMAN PHACO NEEDLE

This author has designed a 700-µm phaco tip made by MicroSurgical Technology (Redmond, WA) to deal with the various issues highlighted previously. It is in standard 30-degree-bevel Kelman (Alcon) conformation with a 20-degree angulation of the shaft. The outer diameter of the needle is 700 µm, but the internal diameter is 570 µm. It is available for the INFINITI (Alcon), Stellaris (Bausch & Lomb), and Signature systems (Abbott Medical Optics), and now has a dedicated sleeve for 1.8-mm phaco surgery. The thin shaft allows excellent fluid entry to the eye due to the added room inside the sleeve. Further, the narrow profile and 30-degree bevel permits easy occlusion. Finally, the unrestricted shaft means that clogging is not an issue even with the densest cataracts. This author has found that it cuts very easily because of the thin profile and the Kelman configuration and holds well for chopping.

SIDE-PORT INSTRUMENTS

Leakage is an issue in surgery through smaller incisions because less fluid is entering the eye through irrigation. If this is not recognized, and often it is not, then anterior chamber stability may be compromised. In order to minimize the side-port leakage, this author has designed a double-ended side-port instrument made by Duckworth & Kent called the Fat Boy chopper (Figure 10-4). One end has a blunt manipulator and the other a sharp vertical chopper. The shaft in the side port is designed to be the same diameter as the custom-designed bimanual irrigation/aspiration handpieces.

IRRIGATION AND ASPIRATION

Bimanual irrigation and aspiration of cortical material seems to be the most efficient method of its removal. Some years ago, in a quest to remove reusable lumens from the surgery practiced in the Eye Unit in Windsor, England, custom-designed bimanual irrigation and aspiration handpieces were introduced (Figure 10-5). The shaft thickness is 20 gauge, which is the same as that of the Fat Boy chopper. The irrigation flow through the handpiece is high at 60 cc/min and anterior chamber stability is good.

LENSES FOR SUB-2-MM COAXIAL MICROINCISIONAL CATARACT SURGERY

Although there have been a variety of plate haptics lenses available for these smaller incisions from ThinOptiX (now discontinued) and Acri.Tec, this author prefers to use 2 other lenses for this surgery. Both need to be injected using a wound-assisted technique. The Akreos MI60 has recently been introduced by Bausch & Lomb and is made from a hydrophilic acrylic with 4 compound haptics. This lens is easily injected through a 1.8-mm incision using the disposable injector provided (Figure 10-6).

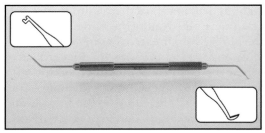

Figure 10-4. Fat Boy chopper. (Reprinted with permission from Duckworth & Kent, Hertfordshire, England.)

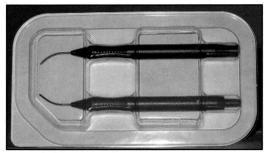

Figure 10-5. Core surgical bimanual irrigation/aspiration.

Figure 10-6. Akreos MI60 intraocular lens. (Reprinted with permission from Bausch & Lomb, Aliso Viejo, CA.)

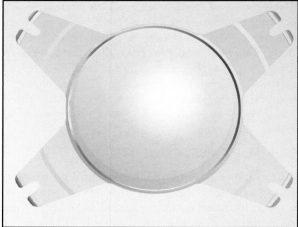

The other lens that can be used is a standard Alcon AcrySof SN60WF IQ. This can either be inserted with the D cartridge using either the Monarch III injector (Alcon) or the Duckworth & Kent single-handed injector. For the former, a 3-handed approach is used, where the surgeon holds the cartridge against the eye and provides countertraction through the side port while the scrub nurse turns the screw on the injector. It provides a very stable injection platform. The Duckworth & Kent injector is used with the surgeon providing side-port countertraction. It is important not to use too much pressure so that the lens does not shoot into the eye.

Questions have been asked about whether significant wound stretching that might impair closure would occur by implanting a full optic lens through these small incisions. This author has presented data on wound measurement before and after implantation of both IOLs that show no more than 0.1-mm change from the end of phacoemulsification.[6]

PHACODYNAMICS FOR SUB-2-MM COAXIAL MICROINCISIONAL CATARACT SURGERY

It is not possible to generalize about machine settings for this microincisional surgery because there are too many variables, such as the following:

* The machine and pump in use
* The phaco tip internal diameter

* The nuclear removal technique used
* The experience of the surgeon
* The hardness of the cataract

These will, as in all phaco surgery, determine the settings. Certain points, however, need to be made. First, the essential for the fluidics with these smaller incisions is to achieve balance within the anterior chamber so that the removal of fluid and lens material and leakage do not destabilize it. Second, whichever form of ultrasound energy is used, whether it be OZil on the INFINITI, longitudinal on the Stellaris, or Ellips on the Signature, an awareness of energy use and thermal effects is critical. It is perfectly possible to set any modern phaco machine to minimize tip temperature rise during surgery even with dense cataracts. This, of course, is helped when mechanical means of disassembling the nucleus like chopping are used in conjunction with appropriate fluidics settings.

SUMMARY

It is now possible for any surgeon to undertake sub-2-mm C-MICS. There are certain salient points to bear in mind that will enhance easy adoption:

* Good and appropriately sized wound construction
* Capsulorrhexis through smaller incisions
* Understanding fluidics balance with lowered irrigation input
* Sensible power modulation
* Wound-assisted insertion techniques

REFERENCES

1. Agarwal A, Agarwal S, Agarwal A, Narang P, Narang S. Phakonit: phacoemulsification through a 0.9 mm corneal incision. *J Cataract Refract Surg.* 2001;27(10):1548-1552.
2. Agarwal A, Agarwal S, Agarwal A. Phakonit with an AcriTec IOL. *J Cataract Refract Surg.* 2003;29(4):854-855.
3. Pandey SK, Wener L, Agarwal A, et al. Phakonit: cataract removal through a sub 1.0 mm incision with implantation of the ThinOptX rollable IOL. *J Cataract Refract Surg.* 2002;28(9):1710-1713.
4. Agarwal A, Trivedi RH, Jacob S, Agarwal A, Agarwal S. Microphakonit: 700 micron cataract surgery. *Clin Ophthalmol.* 2007;1(3):323-325.
5. Agarwal A, Kumar DA, Jacob S, Agarwal A. In vivo analysis of wound architecture in 700 microm microphakonit cataract surgery. *J Cataract Refract Surg.* 2008;34(9):1554-1560.
6. Packard R. Microcoaxial phaco using 1.8 mm incisions: comparison of two machines and IOL systems. Poster presentation at: ASCRS Symposium on Cataract, IOL and Refractive Surgery; April 4-9, 2008; Chicago, IL.

CHAPTER 11

Three-Port Bimanual Sleeveless Microphacoemulsification Using the "Tilt and Tumble" Technique

*Dennis C. Lu, MD; Elizabeth A. Davis, MD;
David R. Hardten, MD; and Richard L. Lindstrom, MD*

The concept of phacoemulsification by Dr. Charles Kelman heralded the era of modern cataract extraction and paved the way for small-incision surgery.[1] The evolution from the large-incision extracapsular cataract extraction, wherein the lens is removed en bloc, to the small incision required by phacoemulsification has led to quicker visual recovery with less induced astigmatism.[2,3] Further reduction in size of the incision would allow for improved safety intraoperatively by providing a more stable anterior chamber and improved safety postoperatively with more rapid wound healing and less risk of endophthalmitis.[4] Furthermore, smaller incisions may accelerate visual rehabilitation.

Currently, reduction in the size of the incision has been limited by the phacoemulsification probe and, in particular, the irrigation sleeve, which requires an incision of at least 2 to 3 mm. Recently, the concept of bimanual sleeveless microphacoemulsification, which has been promoted by Amar Agarwal, MD, has led to the development of sub-1-mm incision phacoemulsification.[5] Intraocular lenses are being developed in order to realize the full benefits of small incision cataract surgery (SICS). At present, the small incisions must be enlarged in order to allow for insertion of the intraocular lens (IOL).[6]

In bimanual microincisional cataract surgery (B-MICS), the large-diameter infusion sleeve is separated from the 0.9- to 1.5-mm titanium phacoemulsification tip, which can then be inserted through a 0.9- to 1.5-mm incision. One of the major concerns of bimanual phacoemulsification is corneal thermal burns from the sleeveless phaco tip.[7] Thus, the fluidics must be optimized to (1) maintain fluid flow through the phaco tip in order to prevent corneal wound burn and (2) maintain a stable anterior chamber during surgery. Additionally, the phacoemulsification settings must be optimized to prevent continuous phacoemulsification from causing excessive heat transfer. This is typically done by cycling the ultrasound on and off with the computer software in the phacoemulsification machine.

In order to maintain a stable anterior chamber, the fluidics must be balanced such that the outflow is equilibrated by inflow. The inflow of fluid in current phacoemulsification units is provided by the infusion sleeve of the phacoemulsification handpiece, which also serves to protect the cornea from thermal injuries. With microphacoemulsification, the infusion sleeve is removed, and irrigation is provided by a second instrument via a paracentesis port. Various irrigating second instruments, such as irrigating choppers and nucleus rotators, are being developed that allow surgeons to continue phacoemulsification using techniques with which they are accustomed. Current irrigating second instruments incorporate 19- to 21-gauge irrigation devices[8] and are typically sufficient to maintain a stable anterior chamber. When the outflow exceeds the inflow, however, an unstable anterior chamber may occur. The concept of 3-port phakonit was devised to reduce the potential of an unstable anterior chamber. A third port allows the insertion of an anterior chamber maintainer that provides additional inflow and thus stabilizes the anterior chamber.[9] This concept is analogous to 3-port vitrectomy, where one port is used for the vitrectomy handpiece, a second port is used for the light pipe, and the third port is used for the infusion device.

TILT AND TUMBLE PHACOEMULSIFICATION

Many of the standard phacoemulsification techniques may be adapted to incorporate microphacoemulsification. The surgeon must be comfortable working through 2 small paracentesis ports and be able to work with both hands equally. Furthermore, the size of the microincision impedes use of traditional capsulorrhexis forceps. Thus, the capsulorrhexis may be accomplished with a needle, cystitome, or specially designed capsulorrhexis forceps.[10]

We will describe the technique of tilt and tumble, which is a form of supracapsular phacoemulsification,[11] and how it is modified to incorporate 3-port bimanual small-incision phacoemulsification. In this technique, the superior pole of the nucleus is tilted above the capsule upon completion of a large capsulorrhexis. Phakonit is then performed while supporting the lens in the iris plane with an irrigating nucleus rotator.

Because tilt and tumble is a supracapsular technique, the risk of endothelial trauma from the instruments or the cataract itself exists. Furthermore, with phakonit, the endothelium in the region of the wound is also at risk of damage from transmitted ultrasound energy by the sleeveless ultrasound probe. Thus, the technique of tilt and tumble is to be used selectively in cases in which there is a relatively deep anterior chamber and a modestly dense cataract. Because a deep anterior chamber is essential to this technique, the inflow provided by current 20-gauge irrigating second instruments may not be sufficient. An anterior chamber maintainer inserted through a third paracentesis may better ensure a deep and stable anterior chamber. Additional protection to the endothelium may be provided by use of a dispersive viscoelastic such as Viscoat (Alcon, Fort Worth, TX) prior to phacoemulsification. Eyes that have shallow anterior chambers, low endothelial cell counts, or very dense nuclei should be approached via an endocapsular technique.

There are several distinct advantages to the tilt and tumble technique. First, it is easy to learn or teach. It is also quick to perform, thus decreasing surgical time. Risk of capsular rupture may be decreased by working in the iris plane. Stress on the zonules is lessened by working out of the bag, making this technique advantageous in cases of pseudoexfoliation. A large capsulorrhexis is required and this virtually eliminates development of a capsular contraction syndrome. However, a large capsulorrhexis may not be appropriate for newer intraocular lenses such as the Alcon ReStor.[12]

INDICATIONS

The indications for the tilt and tumble phacoemulsification technique are quite broad. Tilt and tumble is especially useful in cases of soft and moderately dense cataracts because ultrasound time is significantly reduced by the nature of the technique itself. Because of the use of less phaco energy, this technique is well suited for microphacoemulsification. For example, no grooving is required as in the divide-and-conquer technique. Rather, for moderately dense cataracts, the soft cortical and epinuclear material can be "stripped" with high vacuum interspersed with short pulses of ultrasound. The remaining nugget of nucleus is now substantially reduced in size and can then be phacoemulsified and disassembled at the iris plane. Tilt and tumble also works well for softer cataracts, which are often difficult to split or chop and are also difficult to impale and maneuver. By contrast, in tilt and tumble, tilting the cataract allows one to easily impale and maneuver the superior pole.

This technique can also be utilized in either large or small pupil situations. Some surgeons favor this technique with small pupils because the superior pole of the nucleus can be tilted through the small pupil and can then be safely emulsified above the iris plane. It does require a larger continuous tear anterior capsulectomy of at least 5.0 mm. If a small anterior capsulectomy is achieved, the hydrodissection step of tilting the nucleus can be dangerous, and it is possible to rupture the posterior capsule during the hydrodissection step. If, inadvertently, a small anterior capsulectomy is created, it is probably safest to convert to an endocapsular phacoemulsification technique or enlarge the capsulorrhexis. If it is not possible to tilt the nucleus with either hydrodissection or a manual technique, the surgeon should convert to an endocapsular approach. Occasionally the entire nucleus will subluxate into the anterior chamber. In this setting, if the cornea is healthy, the anterior chamber deep, and the nucleus soft, the phacoemulsification can be completed in the anterior chamber, supporting the nucleus away from the corneal endothelium. The nucleus can also be pushed back inferiorly over the capsular bag to allow the iris plane tilt and tumble technique to be completed.

In patients with severely compromised endothelium, such as Fuchs' dystrophy or previous keratoplasty, and in patients with a low endothelial cell count, endocapsular phacoemulsification is preferred to reduce endothelial stress. In a normal eye, corneal clarity on the first day postoperatively is excellent. Nevertheless, the tilting and tumbling maneuvers do increase the chance of endothelial cell contact with lens material compared to an endocapsular phacoemulsification. Therefore, the endocapsular technique should be employed in eyes with borderline corneas. The technique is a good transition technique for teaching residents, fellows, and surgeons who are transitioning to phacoemulsification because it is easy to convert to a planned extracapsular cataract extraction with the nucleus partially subluxated above the anterior capsular flap at the iris plane.

PREOPERATIVE PREPARATION

The preoperative preparation is no different when adapting tilt and tumble to a bimanual sleeveless microphacoemulsification technique. The patient enters the anesthesia induction or preoperative area and tetracaine drops are placed in both eyes. The placement of these drops increases the patient's comfort during the placement of the multiple dilating and preoperative medications, decreases blepharospasm, and also increases the corneal penetration of the drops to follow.

The eye is dilated with neosynephrine and cyclopentolate. Additionally, preoperative topical antibiotic and anti-inflammatory drops are administered at the same time as the dilating drops. We favor the combination of a preoperative topical antibiotic, topical steroid, and topical nonsteroidal. The rationale for this is to preload the eye with antibiotic and nonsteroidal prior to surgery. The pharmacology of these drugs and the pathophysiology of postoperative infection and inflammation support this approach. An eye that is preloaded with anti-inflammatory drops prior to the surgical insult is likely to have a reduced postoperative inflammatory response. Both topical steroids and nonsteroidals have been found to be synergistic in the reduction of postoperative inflammation. In addition, the use of perioperative antibiotics is supported in the literature as reducing the small chance of postoperative endophthalmitis.[13] Because the patient will be sent home with the same drops utilized preoperatively, there is no additional cost.

Our usual anesthesia is topical tetracaine reinforced with intraoperative intracameral 1% nonpreserved (methylparaben free) lidocaine. For patients with blepharospasm, a facial nerve block utilizing lidocaine can be quite helpful in reducing squeezing of the lids. This block lasts 30 to 45 min and makes surgery easier for the patient and the surgeon. Patients are sedated prior to the block to eliminate any memory of discomfort. One way to determine when this facial nerve block might be useful is to ask the technicians to make a note in the chart when they have difficulty performing applanation pressures or A-scan because of blepharospasm. In these patients, a facial nerve block can be quite helpful.

In younger, anxious patients and in those with difficulty cooperating, we perform a peribulbar or retrobulbar block. Naturally, general anesthesia is used for uncooperative patients and children. Though this is controversial, in some patients where general anesthesia is chosen and a significant bilateral cataract is present, we will perform consecutive bilateral surgery while completely reprepping and starting with fresh instruments for the second eye. Again, this is a clinical decision weighing the risk-to-benefit ratio of operating both eyes on the same day versus the risk of undergoing general anesthesia twice.

Upon entering the surgical suite, the patient table is centered on preplaced marks so that it is appropriately placed for microscope, surgeon, scrub nurse, and anesthetist access. We favor a wrist rest, and the patient's head is adjusted such that a ruler placed on the forehead and cheek will be parallel to the floor. The patient's head is stabilized with tape to the head board to reduce unexpected movements, particularly if the patient falls asleep during the procedure and suddenly awakens. A second drop of tetracaine is placed in each eye. If the tetracaine is placed in each eye, blepharospasm is reduced. A periocular prep with 5% povidone-iodine solution is completed.

An aperture drape is helpful for topical anesthesia to increase comfort. We have noted that when the drape is tucked under the lids, this often irritates the patient's eye and reduces the malleability of the lids, decreasing exposure. Because it is important to isolate the meibomian glands and lashes, a reversible solid-bladed speculum may be used. With temporal and nasal approaches to the eye, the solid blades of the speculum are not in the way. In those cases where a superior approach is planned, a Tegaderm drape (3M, St. Paul, MN) is used and is tucked under the lids. Nevertheless, we have been using a superior approach incision less and less.

Balanced salt solution (BSS) is used in all cases. For the short duration of a phacoemulsification case, BSS plus typically does not provide any clinically meaningful benefit. We place 0.5 cc of the intracardiac nonpreserved (sodium bisulfate free) epinephrine in the bottle for assistance in dilation and perhaps hemostasis. We also add 1 mL (1000 units) of heparin sulfate to reduce the possibility of postoperative fibrin. This is also a good anti-inflammatory and coating agent. At this dose, there is no risk of enhancing bleeding or reducing hemostasis.

A final drop of tetracaine is placed in the operative eye or the surface is irrigated with the nonpreserved lidocaine. We do not like to utilize more than 3 drops of tetracaine or other topical anesthetic because excess softening of the epithelium can occur, resulting in punctate epithelial keratitis, corneal erosion, and delayed postoperative rehabilitation.

Adapting to Bimanual Sleeveless Microphacoemulsification

New skills must be learned and several alterations in technique must be made when modifying the tilt and tumble technique or any other technique to incorporate bimanual sleeveless microphacoemulsification:

* Three 1-mm stab incisions are made to allow for the sleeveless phaco probe, the irrigating second instrument, and the anterior chamber maintainer.
* Because the smaller incision cannot accommodate current capsulorrhexis forceps, we prefer the use of a cystitome to perform the capsulorrhexis. New designs for micro-incisional capsulorrhexis forceps have recently been developed but typically require a steeper learning curve.
* The instruments will behave as if they are "oar-locked" by the small incisions, and thus the surgeon must adapt to reduced mobility of the instruments.[10]
* The skill that is probably most foreign to ophthalmologists is learning how to use the irrigating second instrument and learning how to use the irrigation itself as a tool.[8] Because the irrigating second instrument is no longer coaxial with the phaco probe, it may be used to drive material toward the phaco tip rather than away from the tip as in coaxial irrigation sleeves. An irrigating second instrument can also be used for flipping the epinucleus.[8] In addition, the irrigation may be used to drive the iris away from the phaco tip as in pseudoexfoliation cases with small pupils.
* Microphacoemulsification is a truly bimanual procedure where the instruments may be interchanged between any of the incisions. For example, removal of subincisional cortex may be accomplished by interchanging the irrigating and aspirating handpieces in order to obtain better access to the cortical material. Similarly, interchanging the phaco probe and the irrigating second instrument may be necessary in certain situations, such as in cases of zonular dialysis where traction may be relieved by interchanging the instruments. Consequently, right-handed surgeons must learn how to perform phaco with the left hand and left-handed surgeons must learn how to perform phaco with the right hand.

Operative Procedure

INCISIONS

The patient is asked to look down. The globe is supported with a dry Merocel sponge (Medtronic, Minneapolis, MN), and a counterpuncture is performed superiorly at 12 o'clock with a 1-mm diamond stab knife (Figure 11-1). Approximately 0.25 mL of 1% nonpreserved methylparaben-free lidocaine is injected into the eye. We advise the patient that he or she will feel a tingling or burning for a second, and then the eye will go numb. This provides psychological support for the patient to know that he or she will now have a totally anesthetized eye and should not anticipate any discomfort. We tell our patients that though they will feel some touch and fluid on the eye, they will not feel anything sharp, and if they do, we can supplement the anesthesia.

Two additional stab incisions of approximately 1 mm in width are created in clear cornea for insertion of the phaco probe and the anterior chamber maintainer. The stab incision for the anterior chamber maintainer is placed inferiorly at 6:00. For the phaco probe, we perform a temporal or nasal clear corneal incision just anterior to the vascular arcade and in a direction that is parallel to the iris plane. The direction of this incision prevents an excessively long tunnel and thereby minimizes oar-locking but is shelved enough to

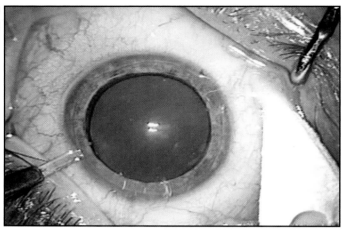

Figure 11-1. Paracentesis port of 1.0 mm is created with a diamond stab knife.

be self-sealing.[8] Incision size is critical in bimanual phacoemulsification because a large incision compromises anterior chamber stability and a small incision causes oar-locking of the instruments. Care is taken not to incise the conjunctiva because this can result in ballooning during the procedure. Some surgeons define this as being a posterior clear corneal incision and others as an anterior limbal incision. The anatomical landmark is the perilimbal capillary plexus and the insertion of the conjunctiva. When the incision is made, there will be a small amount of capillary bleeding. Because the incision is placed into a vascular area, long-term wound healing can be expected to be stronger than it is with a true clear corneal incision. True clear corneal incisions, such as performed in radial keratotomy, clearly do not have the wound-healing capabilities compared to that of a limbal incision where there are functioning blood vessels present.

In right eyes, the incision that we use in the majority of the phakonit cases is temporal, and in left eyes, nasal. This allows the surgeon to sit in the same position for right and left eyes. The nasal cornea is thicker, has a higher endothelial cell count, and allows good access for phacoemulsification. The nasal limbus is approximately 0.3 mm closer to the center of the cornea than the temporal limbus, and this can, in some cases where there is excess edema, reduce first-day postoperative vision more than one might anticipate with a temporal incision. In some patients, there can also be pooling of irrigating fluid, but this problem is less likely in microphacoemulsification where the incisions are more watertight. An aspirating speculum may be useful in situations of pooling. It is also helpful to tip the head slightly to the left side. Nonetheless, in left eyes, a nasal clear corneal approach is an excellent option, particularly for surgeons who find the left temporal position uncomfortable.

Because the incisions are 1 mm, they are almost always self-sealing and do not require a suture unless oar-locking of the instruments stretches the incisions. If stretching of the wounds does occur, the incisions may need to be hydrated to prevent a wound leak. Furthermore, the 1-mm microincisions do not induce astigmatism, whereas incisions of 3 mm in length tend to cause an induction of 0.25 ± 0.25 diopters of astigmatism. In patients with corneal astigmatism, an intraoperative limbal relaxing incision (LRI) can be performed. This can be done at the beginning of the operation. The patient's astigmatism axis is marked to delineate the steep axis of astigmatism. Various LRI nomograms are available to aid the surgeon in determining the magnitude and placement of the arcuate incision. One of the most widely used nomograms was devised by Louis "Skip" Nichamin. The Nichamin Age Adjusted and Pachymetry Adjusted (NAPA) nomogram is unique in that the accuracy is increased due to its adjustment for pachymetry. With this nomogram, the blade depth should be adjusted to 90% peripheral corneal thickness at the planned LRI location. There is an increased variability in response to astigmatic correction with the LRI compard to the excimer laser, but it is unusual to have significant induced astigmatism or wound-related complications with this approach. The outcome goal is a half diopter or less of astigmatism in the preoperative axis. It is preferable to undercorrect rather than overcorrect. The key in astigmatism surgery is "axis, axis, axis." If the incision is placed more than 30 degrees off-axis, the astigmatic result of the LRI is nullified. It is also important not to cross your astigmatic incisions with any of the limbal incisions, which may cause instability and excess ectasia in the area of the incisions.

The anterior chamber is then constituted with a viscoelastic. A dispersive viscoelastic may provide protection to the endothelium. Ocucoat (Bausch & Lomb, Aliso Viejo, CA) has proved be an excellent viscoelastic and can also be utilized to coat the epithelial surface during surgery. This eliminates the need for continuous irrigation with BSS. It gives a very clear view and is also economically a good choice in most settings. Amvisc Plus (Bausch & Lomb) also works well.

CAPSULORRHEXIS

Next, a relatively large-diameter continuous-tear anterior capsulectomy is fashioned. Because the 1-mm incision cannot accommodate traditional capsulorrhexis forceps, the capsulorrhexis may be completed with a cystitome or a bent needle. Alternatively, the surgeon may learn how to use the newer forceps specifically designed for microincisional phacoemulsification. The optimal size of the capsulorrhexis is 5.0 to 5.5 mm in diameter and inside the insertion of the zonules (usually at 7 mm). Larger is typically better than smaller in the tilt and tumble technique because a larger capsulorrhexis allows the cataract to be more easily prolapsed out of the capsular bag. There is less subcapsular epithelium with a larger capsulorrhexis, which may possibly lower the risk of capsular opacification. On the other hand, some feel that a smaller capsulorrhexis that seals over the edge of the intraocular lens may reduce the chances of posterior capsular opacification.[14] If the capsulorrhexis is larger than the IOL, then the capsule will seal down to the posterior capsule around the loops rather than over the anterior surface of the intraocular lens. Most eyes do extremely well with either approach, yet there is still debate as to whether smaller or larger is preferred.

HYDRODISSECTION

Hydrodissection is then performed utilizing a hydrodissection cannula on a 3-cc syringe filled with BSS. Slow continuous hydrodissection is performed, gently lifting the anterior capsular rim until a fluid wave is seen. At this point, irrigation is continued until the nucleus tilts on one side, up and out of the capsular bag. If one retracts the capsule at approximately the 7:30 position with the hydrodissection cannula, usually the nucleus will tilt superiorly. If it tilts in another position, it is simply rotated until it is facing the incision (Figure 11-2).

During the hydrodissection, we depress the posterior lip of the wound in order to prevent the anterior chamber from becoming too deep, which may cause excessive stress on the zonules or disrupt the posterior capsule. However, with the small incisions of microphacoemulsification, depression of the posterior lip may not be as easy.

The anterior chamber maintainer is then inserted through the inferior paracentesis. We prefer to use an anterior chamber maintainer designed with screw-type threads on the infusion tip in order to secure the device within the paracentesis.

Figure 11-2. The nucleus is rotated to face the incision.

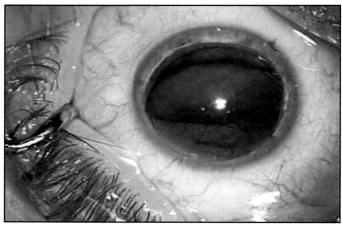

PHACOEMULSIFICATION

Once the nucleus it tilted, additional viscoelastic can be injected under the nucleus, pushing the iris and capsule back. Also, additional viscoelastic can be placed over the nuclear edge to protect the endothelium. A deep anterior chamber is paramount in the tilt and tumble technique. Thus, we prefer using an anterior chamber maintainer inserted through a third port because it provides superior chamber stability over 2-port techniques that rely solely on the irrigation from current 20-gauge irrigating second instruments. The nucleus is then emulsified from outside-in while supporting the nucleus in the iris plane with the irrigating second instrument, such as a nucleus rotator. In order to minimize the use of ultrasound energy, the soft cortical and epinuclear material may be "stripped" with high vacuum interspersed with short bursts of phaco energy. Once half of the nucleus is removed, the remaining half is tumbled upside-down and approached from the opposite pole (Figure 11-3). Again, it is supported in the iris plane until the emulsification is completed (Figure 11-4). Alternatively, the nucleus can be rotated and emulsified from the outside edge in, in a carousel or cartwheel-type of technique. In some cases, the nucleus can be continuously emulsified in the iris plane until the entire nucleus is gone if there is good followability.

This a fast and safe technique and, as mentioned before, it is a modification of the iris plane technique taught by Richard Kratz, MD in the late 1970s and 1980s. It is basically "back to Kratz" with help from Brown and Maloney in the modern phacoemulsification, capsulorrhexis, hydrodissection, and viscoelastic era. Surgery times now range between 5 and 10 min with this approach rather than 10 to 15 min for endocapsular phacoemulsification. In addition, our capsular tear rate has now gone under 1%. Therefore, we find this technique to be easier, faster, and safer. It is true that in this technique, the phacoemulsification tip is closer to the iris margin and also somewhat closer to the corneal endothelium. There is, however, a significantly greater margin of error in regards to the posterior capsule. Care needs to be taken to position the nucleus away from the corneal endothelium and away from the iris margin when utilizing this approach.

If the nucleus does not tilt with simple hydrodissection, it can be tilted with viscoelastic or a second instrument such as a nuclear rotator, Graether collar button (Accutome, Malvern, PA), or hydrodissection cannula.

When utilizing a peristaltic machine, a high flow rate is used, which enhances followability. It is best to maintain a high bottle height in order to maintain a deep anterior chamber, particularly if one chooses to undertake bimanual sleeveless phacoemulsification without an anterior chamber maintainer.

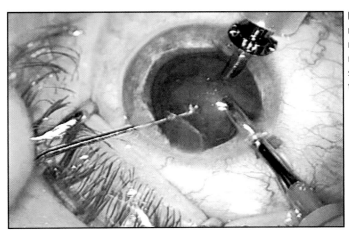

Figure 11-3. The anterior chamber maintainer is inserted into the inferior 1.0-mm paracentesis (3-port microemulsification). The nucleus is supported during phacoemulsification with a second instrument.

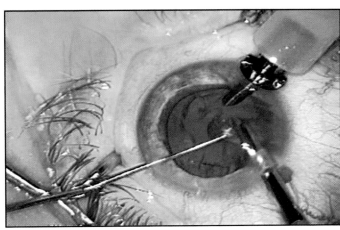

Figure 11-4. Emulsification is completed in the iris plane.

The Dual Linear Millennium (Bausch & Lomb) is also an excellent machine for all cataract techniques including tilt and tumble because it allows the surgeon the choice of either a Venturi pump mode or a peristaltic pump mode. Furthermore, the Millenium's Dual Linear Control is a unique feature that allows for simultaneous control of either flow or vacuum, and ultrasound. In the Venturi pump setting, the foot pedal is arranged such that there is surgeon control over ultrasound on the vertical or pitch motion of the foot pedal, and vacuum control on the yaw or right motion foot pedal. This allows efficient emulsification, and the Millennium is currently our preferred machine. We prefer to set the maximum vacuum in the range of 250 to 300 mm Hg with the bottle height between 120 to 130 cm, which facilitates maintenance of a deep anterior chamber. The maximum ultrasound power is typically set at 60%, with average use of 11% to 15% depending upon the density of the cataract. With the microphacoemulsification technique, we take care to avoid the use of excessive ultrasound power in order to avoid wound burn from the sleeveless phaco tip. In addition, caution must be exercised with higher vacuum levels because it is possible to core through the nucleus and aspirate the iris margin if very high vacuums are utilized.

CORTICAL REMOVAL

Following completion of nuclear removal, the cortex is removed with bimanual irrigation and aspiration. In the absence of an anterior chamber maintainer, the irrigating second instrument may provide irrigation through the paracentesis port while the aspiration device is inserted through the main incision. In the presence of an anterior chamber maintainer, however, irrigation from the second instrument is not necessary. Cortical and epinuclear removal is then performed in the usual manner. For subincisional cortical material, the irrigation and aspiration devices may be interchanged through their respective incisions in order to gain better access. If there is significant debris or plaque on the posterior capsule, one can attempt some polishing and vacuum cleaning, but not so aggressively as to risk capsular tears. Many times there is an unexpected small burr or sharp defect on the irrigation and aspiration tip, which results in a capsular tear after a case that was otherwise well done.

INTRAOCULAR LENS INSERTION

Although IOLs that can be inserted through small incisions are under development, current IOLs cannot take advantage of microincisional surgery. Thus, one of the stab incisions must be enlarged to allow for insertion of the IOL. Alternatively, a new incision may be created, which ensures a well-constructed self-sealing incision that has not been previously stretched by oar-locked instruments.[10] After the capsular bag is reconstituted with viscoelastic, the intraocular lens is inserted utilizing an injector system. We prefer the 3-piece silicone lenses that are injectable through a 3-mm incision.

Excess viscoelastic is removed with irrigation and aspiration. Pushing back on the intraocular lens and slowly turning the irrigation aspiration to the right and left 2 or 3 times allows a fairly complete removal of viscoelastic under the intraocular lens.

We favor injection of a miotic and tend to prefer carbachol over miochol at this time because it is more effective in reducing postoperative intraocular tension spikes and has a longer duration of action. It is best to dilute the carbachol 5 to 1 or one can obtain an excessively small pupil that results in dark vision for the patient at night for 1 to 2 days. The anterior chamber is then refilled through the counterpuncture and the incision is inspected. If the chamber remains well constituted and there is no spontaneous leak from the incision, wound hydration is not necessary. If there is some shallowing in the anterior chamber and a spontaneous leak, wound hydration is performed by injecting BSS peripherally into the incisions and hydrating it to push the edges together. We suspect that within a few minutes, these clear corneal microincisions seal (much as a laser-assisted in situ keratomileusis flap will stick down) through the negative swelling pressure of the cornea and capillary action. It is important to leave the eye slightly firm at 20 mm Hg or so to reduce the side effects of hypotony and help the internal valve incision to appropriately seal.

At completion of the procedure, another drop of antibiotic, steroid, and nonsteroidal is placed on the eye. Additionally, one drop of an antihypertensive such as levobunolol or brimonidine is applied to reduce postoperative intraocular tension spikes. An additional drop of antibiotic is placed in the eye prior to transporting the patient to the postoperative recovery area.

SUMMARY

The next step in the evolution of phacoemulsification may lie in bimanual microphacoemulsification. As newer and thinner IOL designs arise to take advantage of microincisions, the procedure will most certainly gain in popularity. Many of the current phacoemulsification techniques can be readily adapted to bimanual microincisional surgery, thereby allowing a smooth transition for most surgeons. Microincisional surgery may herald a new era where intraoperative and postoperative complications may be reduced.

Acceptance of these new techniques is likely to be slow until development of the new IOL designs matures. These perpetual advances in cataract surgery will continue to translate into improved safety and ultimately greater patient satisfaction.

Some key points include the following:

* The concept of 3-port phakonit was devised to reduce the potential of an unstable anterior chamber. A third port allows the insertion of an anterior chamber maintainer that would provide additional inflow and thus stabilize the anterior chamber.
* This concept is analogous to 3-port vitrectomy, where one port is used for the vitrectomy handpiece, a second port is used for the light pipe, and the third port is used for the infusion device.
* In the tilt and tumble technique, the superior pole of the nucleus is tilted above the capsule upon completion of a large capsulorrhexis. Phakonit is then performed while supporting the lens in the iris plane with an irrigating nucleus rotator.
* Because the tilt and tumble is a supracapsular technique, the risk of endothelial trauma from the instruments or the cataract itself exists. Furthermore, with phakonit, the endothelium in the region of the wound is also at risk of damage from transmitted ultrasound energy by the sleeveless ultrasound probe. The technique of tilt and tumble is to be used selectively in cases in which there is a relatively deep anterior chamber and a modestly dense cataract.
* A deep anterior chamber is essential to this technique and the inflow provided by current 20-gauge irrigating second instruments may not be sufficient. An anterior chamber maintainer inserted through a third paracentesis may better ensure a deep and stable anterior chamber.
* If the nucleus does not tilt with simple hydrodissection, it can be tilted with viscoelastic or a second instrument such as a nuclear rotator, Graether collar button, or hydrodissection cannula.

REFERENCES

1. Kelman CD. Symposium: phacoemulsification. History of emulsification and aspiration of senile cataracts. *Trans Am Acad Ophthalmol Otolaryngol.* 1974;78(1):OP5-OP13.
2. Richards SC, Brodstein RS, Richards WL, Olson RJ, Combe PH, Crowell KE. Long-term course of surgically induced astigmatism. *J Cataract Refract Surg.* 1988;14(3):270-276.
3. Werblin TP. Astigmatism after cataract extraction: 6-year follow up of 6.5- and 12-millimeter incisions. *Refract Corneal Surg.* 1992;8(6):448-458.
4. Tsuneoka H, Shiba T, Takahashi Y. Feasibility of ultrasound cataract surgery with a 1.4 mm incision. *J Cataract Refract Surg.* 2001;27(6):934-940.
5. Agarwal A, Agarwal A, Agarwal S, Narang P, Narang S. Phakonit: phacoemulsification through a 0.9 mm corneal incision. *J Cataract Refract Surg.* 2001;27(10):1548-1552.
6. Tsuneoka H, Hayama A, Takahama M. Ultrasmall-incision bimanual phacoemulsification and AcrySof SA30AL implantation through a 2.2 mm incision. *J Cataract Refract Surg.* 2003;29(6):1070-1076.
7. Braga-Mele R, Liu E. Feasibility of sleeveless bimanual phacoemulsification with the Millennium microsurgical system. *J Cataract Refract Surg.* 2003;29(11):2199-2203.
8. Ifft D. Bimanual microincision phaco. *Ophthalmol Manag.* 2003 Nov:45-56.
9. Agarwal A, Agarwal S, Agarwal A. Phakonit and laser phakonit-cataract surgery through a 0.9-mm incision. In Agarwal S, Agarwal A, Agarwal A, eds. *Phako, Phakonit, and Laser Phako.* El Dorado, Panama: Highlights of Ophthalmology International; 2002.
10. Ronge L. Step-by-step guide to micro phaco. *Eye Net.* 2004;8:23-26.
11. Davis EA, Lindstrom RL. Tilt and tumble phacoemulsification. *Dev Ophthalmol.* 2002;34:44-58.
12. Colvard M. Moving forward with the Crystalens. *Rev Ophthalmol.* 2004. Available at: http://www.revophth.com/index.asp?page=1_453.htm. Accessed January 25, 2010.

13. Soto AM, Mendivil MP. The effect of topical povidone-iodine, intraocular vancomycin, or both on aqueous humor cultures at the time of cataract surgery. *Am J Ophthalmol.* 2001;131(3):293-300.
14. Hollick EJ, Spalton DJ, Meacock WR. The effect of capsulorhexis size on posterior capsular opacification: one-year results of a randomized prospective trial. *Am J Ophthalmol.* 1999;128(3):271-279.

CHAPTER 12

NO-ANESTHESIA SUB-1-MM (700-μM) MICROINCISIONAL CATARACT SURGERY——MICROPHAKONIT

Athiya Agarwal, MD, DO; Soosan Jacob, MS, FRCS, FERC, Dip NB; and Amar Agarwal, MS, FRCS, FRCOphth

On August 15, 1998, Amar Agarwal performed 1-mm cataract surgery by a technique called *phakonit* (phako done with a needle incision technology).[1-13] Dr. Jorge Alio (Spain) coined the term *microincisional cataract surgery*, or MICS,[14] for all surgeries, including laser cataract surgery and phakonit. Dr. Randall Olson first used a 0.8-mm phaco needle and a 21-gauge irrigating chopper and called it *microphaco*.[15-18] On May 21, 2005, a 0.7-mm phaco needle tip with a 0.7-mm irrigating chopper was used for the first time to remove cataracts through the smallest incision possible as of now. This is called *microphakonit*.

NO-ANESTHESIA CATARACT SURGERY

Amar Agarwal was operating a patient with a posterior polar cataract. In such cases, we normally prefer to do an extracapsular cataract extraction under pinpoint anesthesia or subtenons. When he reached the theater, he saw the patient and decided to do phaco; only in the middle of surgery did he realize that no topical anesthetics were applied. On June 13, 1998, he was in Ahmedabad, India, for a live surgery for a workshop organized by the Indian Intraocular Implant and Refractive Society. He decided to do the live surgery without any anesthetic drops. The surgery went very well and there were about 250 eye doctors from all over India watching the surgery. Later a study was done by us that was subsequently published in the *Journal of Cataract and Refractive Surgery*.[19]

FIRST LIVE SURGERY OF PHAKONIT

On August 22, 1998, Amar Agarwal had to do a live surgery in Pune, India, for the Indian Intraocular Implant and Refractive Society conference. He then performed the first live surgery of phakonit. The surgery was done under no anesthesia with just a needle because there was no irrigating chopper at that time and no refined instruments. The surgery went off very well and there were about 350 ophthalmologists who watched the live surgery.

Microphakonit Needle Tip

When we wanted to go for a 0.7-mm phaco needle we wondered whether the needle would be able to hold the energy of the ultrasound. We gave this problem to Larry Laks from MicroSurgical Technology (Redmond, WA) to work on and he made this special 0.7-mm phaco needle (Agarwal's 700-µm microphakonit needle). As you will understand, if we go from a 0.9-mm phaco needle to a 0.7-mm phaco needle, the speed of the surgery will go down. This is because the aspiration flow rate would be less.

It was decided to solve this problem by working on the wall of the 0.7-mm phaco needle. There is a standard wall thickness for all phaco tips. If we say that the outer diameter is a constant, the resultant inner diameter is an area of the outer diameter minus the area of the wall.

The inner diameter will regulate the flow rate/perceived efficiency (which can be good or bad, depending on how you look at it). In order to increase the allowed aspiration flow rate from what a standard 0.7-mm tip would be, Larry Laks made the walls thinner, thus increasing the inner diameter. This would allow a case to go, speed-wise, closer to the speed when using a 0.9-mm tip (not exactly the same, but closer). With gas-forced infusion it would work very well. We decided to go for a 30-degree tip to make it even better.

Microphakonit Irrigating Chopper

We designed two 20-gauge (0.9-mm) irrigating choppers (Figure 12-1) for phakonit when we used the 0.9-mm needle and irrigating chopper. One is the Agarwal 700-µm irrigating chopper made by MicroSurgical Technology. The opening for the fluid is the end opening. This is incorporated in the Duet system (MicroSurgical Technology). The other is Agarwal's 900-µm irrigating chopper made by Geuder (Heidelberg, Germany). This has 2 openings in the side. Depending on the convenience of the surgeon, the surgeon can decide which design of irrigating chopper he or she would like to use. There are advantages and disadvantages with both types of irrigating choppers. The end-opening chopper has an advantage of more fluid coming out of the chopper. The disadvantage is that there is a gush of fluid, which might push the nuclear pieces away. The advantage of the side-opening irrigating chopper is that there is good control because the nuclear pieces are not pushed away, but the disadvantage is that the amount of fluid coming out is much less. If one is using the side-opening irrigating chopper, one should use an air pump or gas-forced infusion.

MicroSurgical Technology increased flow in their irrigating chopper by removing the flow restrictions incorporated in other irrigating choppers as a by-product of their attachment method. They also had control of incisional outflow by making all of the instruments one size and created a matching knife of the proper size and geometry (Figure 12-2).

When we decided to go smaller and use a 0.7-mm irrigating chopper (Figure 12-3) we decided to go for an end-opening irrigating chopper. The bore of the irrigating chopper was smaller so that the amount of fluid coming out of it would be less and an end-opening chopper would maintain the fluidics better. With gas-forced infusion, we thought we would be able to balance the entry and exit of fluid into the anterior chamber. This has been successful.

We measured the amount of fluid coming out of the various irrigating choppers with and without an air pump (Table 12-1). We also measured the values using the simple aquarium air pump (external gas forced infusion) and the Accurus machine (Alcon, Fort Worth, TX) giving internal gas-forced infusion.

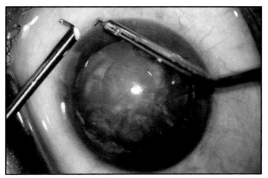

Figure 12-1. Two designs of Agarwal irrigating choppers. The one on the left (700-µm irrigating chopper) has an end opening for fluid. The one on the right (900-µm irrigating chopper) has 2 openings on the sides.

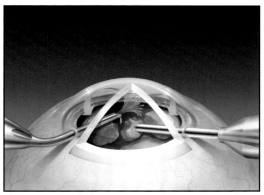

Figure 12-2. Phakonit. Notice the irrigating chopper with an end opening. (Reprinted with permission from MicroSurgical Technology, Redmond, WA.)

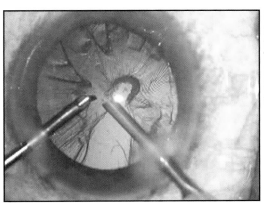

Figure 12-3. Microphakonit. 700-µm irrigating chopper and 700-µm phaco tip without the sleeve inside the eye. All instruments are made by MicroSurgical Technology. The assistant continuously irrigates the phaco probe area from outside to prevent corneal burns. Note that the nucleus has been removed and there are no corneal burns.

Table 12-1

FLUID EXITING FROM VARIOUS IRRIGATING CHOPPERS*

Irrigating Chopper	Without Gas-Forced Infusion	With Gas-Forced Infusion Using the Accurus Machine at 50 mm Hg	With Gas-Forced Infusion Using the Accurus Machine at 75 mm Hg	With Gas-Forced Infusion Using the Accurus Machine at 100 mm Hg	Air Pump With Regulator at Low	Air Pump With Regulator at High
0.9-mm side opening	25	36	42	48	37	51
0.9-mm end opening	34	51	57	65	52	68
0.7-mm end opening	27	39	44	51	41	54

*Values in mL/min.

The 700-μm irrigating chopper that we have designed is basically a sharp chopper that has a sharp cutting edge and helps in karate chopping or quick chopping. It can chop any type of cataract. Table 12-2 shows the differences between coaxial MICS (C-MICS) and bimanual MICS (B-MICS).

Air Pump and Gas-Forced Infusion

The main problem in phakonit was the destabilization of the anterior chamber during surgery. We solved it to a certain extent by using an 18-gauge irrigating chopper. Then Sunita Agarwal suggested the use of an antichamber collapser,[20] which injects air into the infusion bottle. This pushes more fluid into the eye through the irrigating chopper and prevents surge. Thus, we were able to use a 20- to 21-gauge irrigating chopper as well as solve the problem of destabilization of the anterior chamber during surgery. Now, with a 22-gauge (0.7-mm) irrigating chopper, it is essential that gas-forced infusion be used in the surgery. This is also called *external gas-forced infusion*.

When the surgeon uses the air pump contained in the same phaco machine, it is called *internal gas-forced infusion*. To solve the problem of infection, we use a Millipore filter (Billerica, MA) connected to the machine. The Stellaris machine made by Bausch & Lomb (Aliso Viejo, CA) has an inbuilt air pump to give pressurized infusion. When we are using a 0.7-mm irrigating chopper, the problem is that the amount of fluid entering the eye is not enough. To solve this problem, gas-forced infusion is a must. We preset the infusion pump at 100 mm Hg when we are operating using microphakonit.

Bimanual 0.7-mm Irrigation Aspiration System

Bimanual irrigation aspiration is done with the 700-μm bimanual irrigation and aspiration set (MicroSurgical Technology). The previous set we used was the 0.9-mm set. Now with microphakonit, we use the new 0.7-mm bimanual infusion and aspiration set (Figures 12-4 and 12-5) so that we need not enlarge the incision after nucleus removal.

Duet Handles

All of the instruments in the 0.7-mm set fit onto the handles of the Duet system. If a surgeon already has the handles and is using them for phakonit, he or she only needs to get the tips and can use the same handles for microphakonit (Figure 12-6).

Differences Between 0.9-mm and 0.7-mm Sets in Cataract Surgery

Table 12-3 indicates the differences between the 2 techniques.

TECHNIQUE

Incision

The incision is made with a keratome. This can be done using a sapphire knife or a stainless steel knife. One should be careful when one is making the incision so that the incision is a bit long, as if one would be using gas-forced infusion in microphakonit. Before making the incision, a needle with viscoelastic is taken and pierced in the eye in the area where the side port has to be made. The viscoelastic is then injected inside the eye.

Table 12-2

PHACO VERSUS PHAKONIT*

Feature	Phaco	Phakonit (B-MICS)
1. Incision size	3 mm	Sub 1.4 mm
2. Air pump	Not mandatory	Mandatory
3. Hand usage	Single-handed phaco possible	Two hands (bimanual)
4. Nondominant hand entry and exit	Last to enter and first to exit	First to enter and last to exit
5. Capsulorrhexis	Needle or forceps	Better with needle
6. IOL	Foldable IOL	Rollable IOL
7. Astigmatism	Two unequal incisions create astigmatism	Two equal ultrasmall incisions negate the induced astigmatism
8. Stability of refraction	Later than phakonit	Earlier than phaco
9. Iris prolapse—intraoperative	More chances	Less chances due to smaller incision

*C-MICS indicates coaxial microincisional cataract surgery; B-MICS, bimanual microincisional cataract surgery; IOL, intraocular lens.

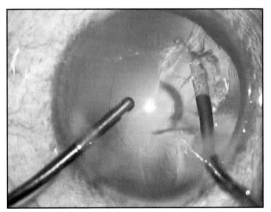

Figure 12-4. Bimanual irrigation aspiration with the 700-µm set.

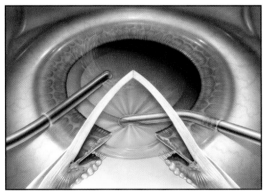

Figure 12-5. Soft-tip irrigation and aspiration. (Reprinted with permission from MicroSurgical Technology, Redmond, WA.)

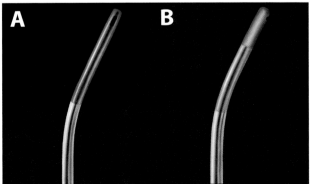

Figure 12-6. 700-µm irrigation aspiration tips. (A) Irrigation tip. (B) Aspiration tip. (Reprinted with permission from MicroSurgical Technology, Redmond, WA.)

Table 12-3

DIFFERENCES BETWEEN PHAKONIT AND MICROPHAKONIT

Features	Phakonit	Microphakonit
Irrigating chopper	0.9 mm	0.7 mm
Phaco needle	0.9 mm	0.7 mm
Control in surgery	Good	Better control
Valve construction	Extremely important	Not important because incision is much smaller
Iris prolapse	Can occur if valve is bad	Very rare
Intraoperative floppy iris syndrome	Can be managed	Much better to manage because incision is much smaller and there is better control
Hydrodissection	Can be done from both incisions	Be careful because very little space is there for escape of fluid
Air pump (GFI)	Can be done without it, but better with it	Mandatory; 0.7-mm irrigating choppers even with higher end machines need GFI
Flow rate	Can keep any value	Do not keep it very high; 20-24 mL/min
Bimanual I/A	0.9 mm	0.7 mm

*GFI indicates gas-forced infusion; I/A, irrigation and aspiration.

This will distend the eye so that the clear corneal incision can be made easily. Make one clear corneal incision between the lateral rectus and inferior rectus and the other between the lateral rectus and superior rectus. In this way, one is able to control the movements of the eye during surgery.

Rhexis

The rhexis of about 5 to 6 mm is then performed. This is done with a needle (Figure 12-7). A straight rod is held in the left hand to stabilize the eye. This is the globe stabilization rod. The advantage of this is that the movements of the eye can be controlled if one is working without any anesthesia or under topical anesthesia. One can also use a microrhexis forceps (Figures 12-8 and 12-9).

HYDRODISSECTION

Hydrodissection is performed and the fluid wave passing under the nucleus is checked. Check for rotation of the nucleus. The advantage of microphakonit is that one can do hydrodissection from both incisions so that even the subincisional areas can be easily hydrodissected. Because there is not much escape of fluid, one should be careful in hydrodissection because if too much fluid is passed into the eye, complications can occur.

MICROPHAKONIT

The 22-gauge (0.7-mm) irrigating chopper connected to the infusion line of the phaco machine is introduced with the foot pedal on position 1. The phaco probe is connected to the aspiration line, and the 0.7-mm phaco tip without an infusion sleeve is introduced

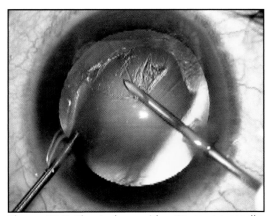

Figure 12-7. Rhexis done with a 26-gauge needle. This has viscoelastic in it so that if the chamber shallows one can inject viscoelastic inside the eye. Note that the other hand has Agarwal's globe stabilization rod (Katena, Denville, NJ).

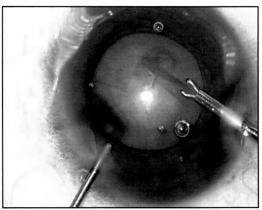

Figure 12-8. MicroSurgical Technology 25-gauge microrhexis forceps used to perform the rhexis in a mature cataract. Note the trypan blue staining the anterior capsule.

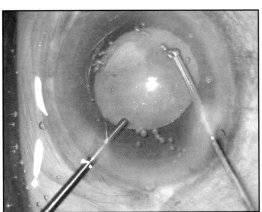

Figure 12-9. 25-gauge microrhexis forceps for sub-1-mm cataract surgery.

through the clear corneal incision. Using the phaco tip with moderate ultrasound power, the center of the nucleus is directly embedded starting from the superior edge of rhexis with the phaco probe directed obliquely downwards toward the vitreous. The settings at this stage are 50% phaco power, flow rate 20 mL/min, and 100 to 200 mm Hg vacuum. Using the karate chop technique, the nucleus is chopped. Thus, the whole nucleus is removed. Cortical washing is then done with the bimanual irrigation and aspiration (0.7-mm set) technique. During the entire microphakonit procedure, gas-forced infusion is used.

Summary

With microphakonit, a 0.7-mm set is used to remove the cataract. At present, this is the smallest one can use for cataract surgery. With time, one would be able to go smaller with better instruments and devices. The problem at present is the intraocular lens (IOL). We have to get good quality IOLs going through sub-1-mm cataract surgical incisions so that the real benefit of microphakonit can be given to the patient.

References

1. Agarwal A, Agarwal S, Agarwal A. No anesthesia cataract surgery. In: Agarwal A, Agarwal S, Agarwal A, eds. *Phacoemulsification, Laser Cataract Surgery and Foldable IOLs*. New Delhi, India: Jaypee; 1998:144-154.
2. Pandey SK, Wener L, Agarwal A, Agarwal S, Agarwal A, Apple D. No-anesthesia cataract surgery. *J Cataract Refract Surg*. 2001;28:1710.
3. Agarwal A, Agarwal S, Agarwal A. Phakonit: a new technique of removing cataracts through a 0.9 mm incision. In: Agarwal A, Agarwal S, Agarwal A, eds. *Phacoemulsification, Laser Cataract Surgery and Foldable IOLs*. New Delhi, India: Jaypee; 1998:139-143.
4. Agarwal A, Agarwal S, Agarwal A. Phakonit and laser phakonit: lens surgery through a 0.9 mm incision. In: Agarwal A, Agarwal S, Agarwal A, eds. *Phacoemulsification, Laser Cataract Surgery and Foldable IOL's*. 2nd ed. New Delhi, India: Jaypee; 2000:204-216.
5. Agarwal A, Agarwal S, Agarwal A. Phakonit. In: Agarwal A, Agarwal S, Agarwal A, eds. *Phacoemulsification, Laser Cataract Surgery and Foldable IOL's*. 3rd ed. New Delhi, India: Jaypee; 2003:317-329.
6. Agarwal A, Agarwal S, Agarwal A. Phakonit and laser phakonit. In: Boyd BF, Agarwal S, Agarwal A, Agarwal A, eds. *LASIK and beyond LASIK: Wavefront Analysis and Customized Ablation*. El Dorado, Panama: Highlights of Ophthalmology; 2000:463-468.
7. Agarwal A, Agarwal S, Agarwal A. Phakonit and laser phakonit—cataract surgery through a 0.9 mm incision. In: Boyd BF, Boyd S, eds. *Phako, Phakonit and Laser Phako*. Panama: Highlights of Ophthalmology; 2002:327-334.
8. Agarwal A, Agarwal S, Agarwal A. The phakonit ThinOptX IOL. In: Agarwal A, ed. *Presbyopia*. Thorofare, NJ: SLACK Incorporated; 2002:187-194.
9. Agarwal A, Agarwal S, Agarwal A. Antichamber collapser. *J Cataract Refract Surg*. 2002;28(7):1085-1086.
10. Pandey S, Wener L, Agarwal A, et al. Phakonit: cataract removal through a sub 1.0 mm incision with implantation of the ThinOptX rollable IOL. *J Cataract Refract Surg*. 2002;28(9):1710-1713.
11. Agarwal A, Agarwal S, Agarwal A. Phakonit: phacoemulsification through a 0.9 mm incision. *J Cataract Refract Surg*. 2001;27(10):1548-1552.
12. Agarwal A, Agarwal S, Agarwal A, Narang P, Narang S. Phakonit with an Acritec IOL. *J Cataract Refract Surg*. 2003;29:854-855.
13. Agarwal S, Agarwal A, Agarwal A. *Phakonit With Acritec IOL*. El Dorado, Panama: Highlights of Ophthalmology; 2000.
14. Alío J. What does MICS require. In: Alío J, ed. *MICS*. El Dorado, Panama: Highlights of Ophthalmology; 2004:1-4.
15. Soscia W, Howard JG, Olson RJ. Microphacoemulsification with Whitestar. A wound-temperature study. *J Cataract Refract Surg*. 2002;28(6):1044-1046.
16. Soscia W, Howard JG, Olson RJ. Bimanual phacoemulsification through two stab incisions. A wound-temperature study. *J Cataract Refract Surg*. 2002;28:1039-1043.
17. Olson R. Microphaco chop. In: Chang D, ed. *Phaco Chop*. Thorofare, NJ: SLACK Incorporated; 2004:227-237.
18. Chang D. Bimanual phaco chop. In: Chang D, ed. *Phaco Chop*. Thorofare, NJ: SLACK Incorporated; 2004:239-250.
19. Pandey SK, Werner L, Apple DJ, Agarwal A, Agarwal A, Agarwal S.. No-anesthesia clear corneal phacoemulsification versus topical and topical plus intracameral anaesthesia; randomized clinical trial. *J Cataract Refract Surg*. 2001;27(10):1643-1650.
20. Agarwal A. Air pump. In: Agarwal A, ed. *Bimanual Phaco: Mastering the Phakonit/MICS Technique*. Thorofare, NJ: SLACK Incorporated; 2005.

CHAPTER 13

USE OF BIMANUAL MICS FOR DIFFICULT AND CHALLENGING CASES

I. Howard Fine, MD; Richard S. Hoffman, MD; and Mark Packer, MD, FACS

The advantages of bimanual microincisional cataract surgery (B-MICS) have been elaborated in a variety of papers within the literature.[1-5] We believe the technique has distinct fluidic advantages because by separating inflow from aspiration and phaco, all of the fluid is coming in through one side of the eye and exiting through the opposite side of the eye, so there are never competing currents at the phaco tip. In addition, it is easier to achieve a nearly closed system because of the tightness of the incisions, and we can address certain cases that would be less advantageous, or even impossible, with the use of a coaxial phaco tip.

HIGH MYOPIA

In highly myopic eyes, we are able to achieve a situation in which we can maintain the anterior chamber in a completely stable configuration, never trampolining the vitreous face, by keeping the irrigating handpiece in the eye throughout the case. Chopping can take place in the usual manner, and with the completion of chopping, we can keep the irrigating chopper in the eye, remove the phaco needle, place viscoelastic, remove residual cortex, and then place viscoelastic for the implantation of the intraocular lens (IOL) without ever shallowing the anterior chamber. We believe that there may eventually be a documented decreased incidence of retinal detachment in high myopia as a result of nontrampolining of the vitreous face during phaco and the implantation of IOLs that fill the capsule, such as dual-optic IOLs or IOLs that arch posteriorly, such as the Crystalens (Bausch & Lomb, Aliso Viejo, CA).

POSTERIOR POLAR CATARACT

In the situation of posterior polar cataracts (Figure 13-1), 35% have defective posterior capsules and almost all of them have weakened capsules, so it is important to not overpressurize the eye and perhaps force nuclear material through the defective posterior capsule. By the same token, it is important to not shallow the chamber and have the nucleus come forward and possibly open the defect in the posterior capsule. These cases are advantageously done with bimanual microincision phacoemulsification.

Figure 13-2. Bringing nuclear material out of the posterior chamber with an unsleeved phaco tip in the presence of zonular dialysis.

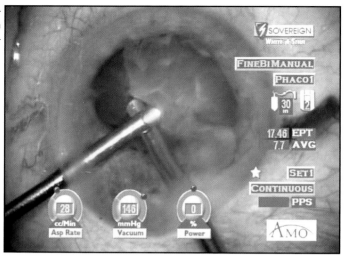

Figure 13-3. Injection of a capsule tension ring through a microincision controlled by a Lester hook in the right hand.

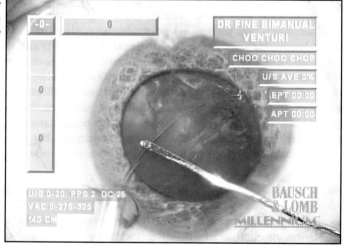

force on the lens that might stress the residual zonules. Cortical cleanup is facilitated in the presence of an endocapsular tension ring by performing gentle cortical cleaving hydrodissection prior to the implantation of the ring. The lens is then implanted into the capsular bag through an incision between the 2 side-port incisions, which is our routine method for IOL implantation in the presence of 2 1.1-mm phacoemulsification incisions.

ROCK-HARD NUCLEI

We can phacoemulsify rock-hard nuclei (Figure 13-4) with the same facility and ease with which we do softer nuclei with bimanual microincision phacoemulsification, and we usually end up with average phaco powers under 10% with effective phaco times under 10 s, in spite of the density of these nuclei. This is an enormous advantage in terms of corneal endothelial protection because of the great stability of the anterior chamber. We prefer a 30-degree phacoemulsification tip used with the bevel down.

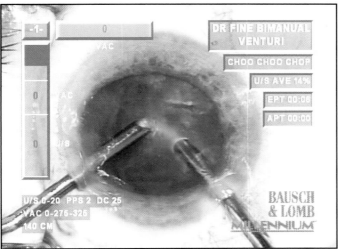

Figure 13-4. Chopping a rock-hard nucleus.

This allows the achievement of vacuum once the tip touches the endonucleus. A bevel-up tip must go deep into the nucleus before occlusion and vacuum are achieved. With a bevel-down tip, we are also sending all of the energy toward the nucleus and none toward the endothelium or trabecular meshwork. Finally, one can mobilize pie-shaped segments from the level of the capsulorrhexis up, rather than having to go deep into the endolenticular space to achieve occlusion to mobilize these segments, as we would have to with a bevel-up configuration.

SWITCHING HANDS

In cases of zonular dialysis, another advantage of B-MICS is that we can use the phaco tip with either hand. After inserting an endocapsular tension ring through one of the microincisions, we would hydroexpress the lens into the plane of the capsulorrhexis and then utilize the phaco tip in either the right or left hand, depending on the zonular dialysis. For dialyses that are on the right side, we would use the phaco tip in the right hand, drawing material in the anterior chamber toward the area of weakened zonules, rather than away from it, which would stress the intact zonules. For dialyses that are on the left-hand side, we can use the phaco tip in our left hand and the irrigating chopper in the right to remove the nucleus, thereby closing the zonular dialysis with the activation of flow and vacuum toward the left side.

MICROCORNEA OR MICROPHTHALMOS

For very small eyes, such as microcornea or microphthalmos, the use of B-MICS is enormously advantageous because the smaller size of the instruments allows us, through 2 clear corneal microincisions, to maintain excellent visualization. A coaxial tip, which is much larger in size, would indent the cornea as it was manipulated and partially obscure the visualization of the intraocular structures. This has turned out to be especially advantageous in cases with a microcornea or a microphthalmic eye in the presence of an unusually large lens.

Postmalignant Melanoma

In one case in which 100 degrees of ciliary body and iris, with the exception of the sphincter, were excised for malignant melanoma (Figure 13-5), we were able to perform B-MICS through 2 microincisions on each side of the 100-degree missing ciliary body and iris. The advantage here is that with the vitreous face open to the anterior chamber, we wanted to be drawing material toward the area of missing zonules after having sequestered the vitreous in that area with sodium hyaluronate (Healon 5). Phacoemulsification performed in other locations would bring vitreous to the phaco tip and provide a much more challenging situation. The IOL was implanted nasally over the intact zonules to force the lens to push against the area of missing zonules, rather than to pull away from the area of missing zonules if it had been implanted in the temporal periphery.

Intraoperative Floppy Iris Syndrome

We find B-MICS enormously useful in cases of intraoperative floppy iris syndrome (IFIS). If we have adequate dilation in the presence of a floppy iris, we will perform gentle cortical cleaving hydrodelineation and hydrodissection and then hydroexpress the lens into the plane of the iris. We will then carousel the endonucleus in the plane of the capsulorrhexis with the irrigating cannula held high in the anterior chamber. Holding the irrigator high in the anterior chamber allows for a tamponading of the iris and disallows floppiness, or billowing, of the iris. After removing the endonucleus in the plane of the capsulorrhexis, we see a fully intact epinuclear shell, which had been sitting on top of the iris, helping to hold it back (Figure 13-6). This is an extremely advantageous technique for nuclei of less hard densities that can be carouselled and phacoed in the anterior chamber without threatening the corneal endothelium.

For harder cataracts, and in the presence of pupils that will not dilate well, we will dilate the pupil with Healon 5, do a rather large capsulorrhexis, and then do one endolenticular chop. We then keep the irrigating chopper high in the anterior chamber and, with the unsleeved phaco tip, bring nuclear material up to the chopper held high in the anterior chamber for further disassembly. This allows, once again, a tamponading of the iris and prevention of billowing or floppiness. We try to keep the phaco needle occluded and in foot position 2 or 3, but with a clearance of occlusion, we go to foot position 1 in order to minimize evacuation of Healon 5, which is holding open the pupil.

After the endonucleus is removed in this way, we remove the epinucleus. Because it is harder to keep the tip occluded with epinuclear trimming and flipping, there tends to be evacuation of Healon 5 and a reduction of the size of the pupil, although because of the irrigator held high in the anterior chamber, it does not billow. We then have to re-instill Healon 5 to redilate the pupil. Then, once again, holding the irrigator high in the anterior chamber, we keep the aspirating microincision handpiece occluded by going circumferentially around the capsulorrhexis, removing the cortical material only from the fornix of the capsule, letting it sit as a cluster in the central portion of the capsule. After all of the cortex has been mobilized from the capsular fornix, we remove the residual cortex from the eye. In this way, we are able to keep Healon 5 in the eye and disallow miosis of the pupil until the case is complete.

Refractive Lens Exchange

We can do refractive lens exchange easily and safely with bimanual microincision phacoemulsification. We do cortical cleaving hydrodissection and no hydrodelineation.

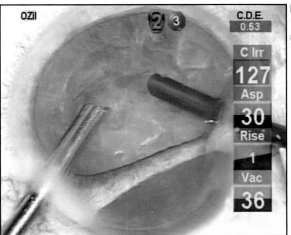

Figure 13-5. Initial chop of the cataract post-100-degree ciliary body excision for malignant melanoma.

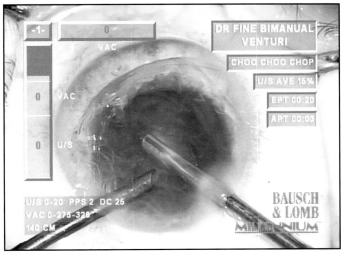

Figure 13-6. Epinucleus holding the iris back after carouselling the endonucleus in the presence of intraoperative floppy iris syndrome.

We then hydroexpress the lens into the plane of the capsulorrhexis and carousel it without any phacoemulsification energy for soft lenses, usually encountered in refractive lens exchange. We do an entirely fluidic-based extraction and then, because of cortical cleaving hydrodissection, we are able to evacuate the cortex by just tilting the phaco tip back into the posterior chamber where it jumps into the phaco tip as a single piece.

REFRACTIVE LENS EXCHANGE IN POSTRADIAL KERATOTOMY

In cases where previous radial keratotomy (RK) has been performed, we can do bimanual microincision clear lens or cataract removal by going between 2 previously placed radials, making it much less likely that we will rupture the radial incisions during the course of the lens extraction. We then make an incision between our 2 microincisions for implantation of the IOL, but in the presence of previous RK, we make it through the posterior limbus for implantation of the IOL (Figure 13-7).

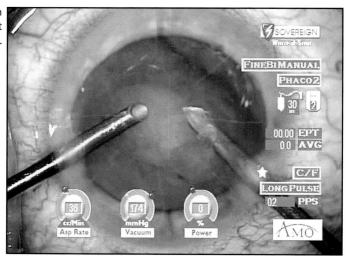

Figure 13-7. Bimanual microincision phacoemulsification of a cataract between radial keratotomy incisions.

INTRAOCULAR CAUTERY

We have found that we can also, with bimanual microincision instruments, do intraocular cautery by using an irrigating cannula in one of the microincisions and a microincision bipolar cautery in the other. Pinching the irrigation tubing allows bleeding to take place, clearly identifying the point source because the eye softens and the bleeding points start to ooze. We cauterize them precisely with the bipolar cautery and therefore minimize trauma to intraocular structures by avoiding more cautery than is necessary.

BIMANUAL MICROINCISION INSTRUMENTS

A number of other instruments have been developed for use through 1.1-mm microincisions. Iris reconstruction is much easier utilizing intraocular forceps that stabilize the iris for suturing. New intraocular needle holders are also usable through a 1.0-mm incision. In this way, fragile and atrophic irides can be sutured without putting excessive stress on the iris tissue. The knots are tied with a Siepser external tying mechanism, and the knots are cut with an intraocular microincision scissors, which are also admissible through a 1.0-mm incision.

For late reopening of capsular bags to recenter IOLs, we can enlarge a capsulorrhexis in the late postoperative period by nicking the rhexis with intraocular scissors and then tearing a larger opening with a microincision capsulorrhexis forceps (Figure 13-8). Viscodissection of the lens within the capsular bag can be accomplished through microincisions, which also allows for repositioning of IOLs without the need to make larger incisions to manipulate them intraocularly. Additional microincision instruments are currently under a state of development, including microincision Colibri forceps, microincision iris graspers (MicroSurgical Technology, Redmond, WA), and microincision intraocular lens holders and cutters (MicroSurgical Technology).

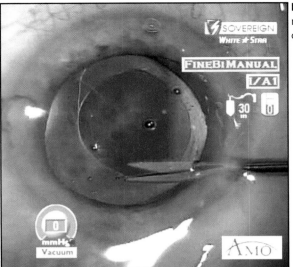

Figure 13-8. Nicking the capsulorrhexis with microincision scissors prior to enlarging the capsulorrhexis.

Summary

We believe that B-MICS is a technique that has a very short learning curve, is highly atraumatic, and is unquestionably the technique of the future. For those who are willing to go through the short learning curve now, it represents the best and safest technique at present for the management of certain difficult and challenging cases.

References

1. Agarwal A, Agarwal A, Agarwal S, Narang P, Narang S. Phakonit: phacoemulsification through a 0.9 mm corneal incision. *J Cataract Refract Surg.* 2001;27(10):1548-1552.
2. Fine IH, Packer M, Hoffman RS. Use of power modulations in phacoemulsification: choo-choo chop and flip phacoemulsification. *J Cataract Refract Surg.* 2001;27(2):188-197.
3. Fine IH. The choo choo chop and flip phacoemulsification technique. *Oper Tech Cataract Refract Surg.* 1998;1:61-65.
4. Fine, IH, Hoffman RS, Packer M. Bimanual microincision phacoemulsification for difficult and challenging cases. Garg A, Alio J, eds. *Surgical Techniques in Ophthalmology: Cataract Surgery.* New Delhi, India: Jaypee Brothers; 2010:Chapter 41.
5. Alio J, Fine IH, eds. *Minimizing Incisions and Maximizing Outcomes in Cataract Surgery.* New York, NY: Springer; 2010.

CHAPTER 14

MICROINCISIONAL CATARACT SURGERY FOR PEDIATRIC CATARACTS

Arturo Pèrez-Arteaga, MD

Microincisional cataract surgery (MICS) was conceived as a minimally invasive technique because of the smaller incisions in comparison to the conventional phaco technique. With time, its use, and continuous implementation, it has finally been demonstrated that this technique is not "a matter of incision size, it is truly a matter of fluidics improvement."[1-3] Microincisional techniques have shown an improvement in wound construction and healing, stability of the globe during phacoemulsification and irrigation/aspiration techniques, and the capability to avoid surge and decrease the amount of total irrigation inside the eye in comparison to standard phacoemulsification technology.

MICROPHAKONIT: 700-MICRON CATARACT SURGERY

700-μm technology (also called *microphakonit* or *micro-bimanual technique*) corresponds to the smallest possible procedure to obtain aphakia (Figure 14-1). All of the advantages of MICS are enhanced when the instruments become smaller, including wound stability, fluidics improvement, and decrease in time of visual recovery in comparison with other techniques.

Because the eye containing a pediatric cataract is small and because the tissues are delicate, management of fluidics is important.[1-10] The nucleus is soft and complete removal of lens matter is mandatory because it has an increased propensity for postoperative inflammation. An anterior vitrectomy is needed to avoid a frequently observed posterior capsule opacification, so 700-μm technology for lens removal is a good choice for these particular cases (Figure 14-2).

CLINICAL FEATURES OF THE PEDIATRIC CATARACT, PREOPERATIVE EVALUATION, AND SURGICAL INDICATIONS

Pediatric cataract poses particular features; for example, an increased tendency toward a posterior capsule opacification.

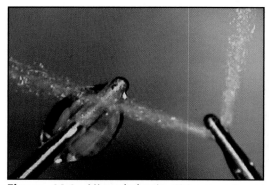

Figure 14-1. Microphakonit 700-μm cataract surgery instruments (MicroSurgical Technology, Redmond, WA).

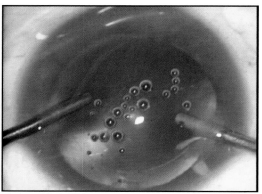

Figure 14-2. 700-μm cataract surgery in a pediatric cataract.

PREOPERATIVE EVALUATION

In all cataract cases, the surgery begins with the preoperative evaluation. However, in cases of pediatric cataract, this concept acquires a major relevance. Every child with cataract should have a thorough systemic history and physical examination by a pediatrician or other qualified specialist (eg, genetics) and laboratory evaluation as indicated based on positive findings. When cataract in childhood is associated with a dysmorphic syndrome or systemic disease, some extraocular abnormality is usually fairly obvious and is evident at the time of diagnosis.

The ophthalmic evaluation process starts with examination of the anterior segment. Some children can be immobilized and others will require sedation or even exploration under anesthesia. Anterior segment characteristics must be addressed; signs of uveitis (sometimes quite subtle) indicate the presence of an underlying disorder such as juvenile rheumatoid arthritis (characterized by the presence of iris-lens synechiae and band keratopathy), Fuchs' heterochromic iridocyclitis, or pars planitis. Corneal diameter needs to be measured or estimated as reliably as possible, searching for megalocornea or congenital glaucoma. The quality of the red fundus reflex must be critically assessed in every child with cataract. This can be done with the direct ophthalmoscope at 30 cm of distance, the best instrument and clinical technique for this purpose. The posterior pole can be assessed by direct or indirect ophthalmoscopy, looking particularly for underdevelopment or malformation of the disc or macula and the presence of abnormal pigmentation; pigmentary retinopathy may be visible in eyes afflicted with rubella or other congenital infection. B-scan ultrasonography is necessary if no fundus view is obtainable, posterior segment malformation can be detected by ultrasonography in some cases of vitreous persistence, and rhegmatogenous retinal detachment occurs in a significant number of patients with cataract caused by atopic dermatitis. Intraocular pressure (IOP) measurement should be done on every eye with a cataract; an elevated IOP may accompany congenital cataract associated with rubella infection or Lowe syndrome. The intraocular lens (IOL) power calculation can be done in the operating room immediately prior to surgery or even transoperative, taking advantage of the anesthesia, through an intraoperative aphakic refraction method.

SURGICAL INDICATIONS

Most polar opacities (particularly those involving only the anterior capsule), smaller nuclear cataracts, and lamellar cortical opacities that transmit light centrally can be left alone and no surgery should be indicated until an age when visual impairment is noticed. Posterior cortical cataracts (especially those resulting from posterior lenticonus) usually do not become visually significant until months or years after birth. A posterior subcapsular cataract (Figure 14-3), if producing loss of vision or amblyopia, should be treated.

ADVANTAGES AND SURGICAL TECHNIQUE OF BIMANUAL MICROINCISIONAL CATARACT SURGERY TECHNOLOGY FOR REMOVAL OF PEDIATRIC CATARACTS

INCISIONS

With the utilization of 700-µm technology for lens removal, 2 incisions should be performed in the clear cornea at the 10 and 2 o'clock meridians. The surgeon must be sure to utilize adequate instrumentation because leakage of the incisions may lead to intraoperative surge, whereas an incision that is too tight can lead to corneal trauma. Some surgeons like to perform the third incision (for IOL implantation) at the beginning because the eye has a better pressure at this time than after the lens removal and because it can function as a third position for instrumentation during some particular maneuvers. The incision for the nondominant hand will be for the irrigating devices, and the incision for the dominant hand will be for the aspirating cannulas, phaco tips, and vitrectors. One can use an anterior chamber maintainer to provide continuous infusion and prevent collapse of the anterior chamber with the 700-µm technique, but if one uses gas-forced infusion, this is not necessary.

ANTERIOR CAPSULE MANAGEMENT

The features of the anterior capsule in the pediatric cataract are different from the adult cataract. Many of the capsules are fibrotic. Others have weak zonular attachments, have a high degree of elasticity, or may not contain any material within the capsular bag. Creation of an adequate opening to the anterior capsule is crucial to enable a complete removal of the lens material. One can use trypan blue to get a good rhexis.

NUCLEAR AND CORTICAL PARTICLES REMOVAL: MASTERING THE FLUIDICS MANAGEMENT AND ANTERIOR CHAMBER STABILITY

After the capsulorrhexis has been created, hydrodissection is the next step. This would make the soft nucleus prolapse out of the bag and this can then be aspirated or emulsified with the 700-µm phaco needle (MicroSurgical Technology). In this particular technique, the irrigating cannula is inserted through the incision for the nondominant hand (no irrigating choppers are needed because the lens material is soft and no chopper maneuvers are needed); the aspirating cannula is inserted through the dominant-hand incision; both cannulas are 0.7 mm. The air pump is kept on during the surgery and for cortical aspiration to prevent any surge.

POSTERIOR CAPSULE MANAGEMENT AND INTRAOCULAR LENS PLACEMENT

The management of the posterior capsule after the complete removal of the lens material is still a source of controversy among pediatric surgeons. Whereas some like to leave it intact as in the adult cataract (either with or without IOL implantation), others like to perform a posterior capsulorrhexis followed by dissection of the anterior hyaloid face or an anterior vitrectomy for IOL implantation with capsular fixation (Figure 14-4).

Figure 14-3. Posterior subcapsular cataract.

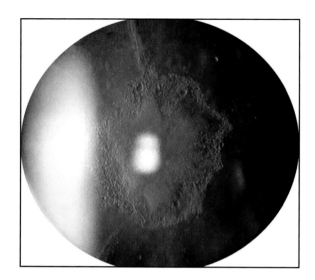

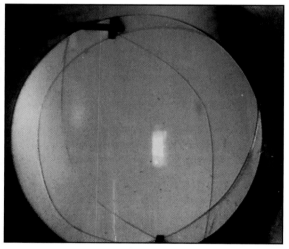

Figure 14-4. Photograph of an eye implanted with an acrylic (AcrySof, Alcon, Fort Worth, TX) intraocular lens (IOL) in the capsular bag. IOL optic capture through a posterior capsulorrhexis was performed during the primary procedure. This photograph was taken at 1 month postoperatively and shows a well-centered IOL and anterior and posterior capsulorrhexis edges. (Reprinted with permission from Pandey SK, Wilson E. Principles and paradigms of pediatric cataract surgery and intraocular lens implantation. In: Agarwal A, ed. *Phaco Nightmares: Conquering Cataract Catastrophes*. Thorofare, NJ: SLACK Incorporated; 2006:65-98.)

Precipitates composed of pigments, inflammatory cells, fibrin, blood breakdown products, and other elements are often seen during the immediate postoperative period on the surface of an IOL optic implanted in a child (Figure 14-5). The deposits can be pigmented or nonpigmented but are usually not visually significant. They occur much more commonly in children with dark irises and when compliance with postoperative medications has been poor. Heparin-surface-modified IOLs have been reported to decrease the incidence of these deposits.

BIMANUAL ANTERIOR VITRECTOMY

Vitrectomy in the pediatric cataract may be planned or unplanned. Because the perils of leaving behind residual lens material are well recognized, surgeons attempt to achieve nearly complete removal of the lens, found in the automated vitrector, ideally suited for this purpose. We believe that if an anterior vitrectomy is performed, it has to be done with a biaxial approach, as the entire procedure was done.

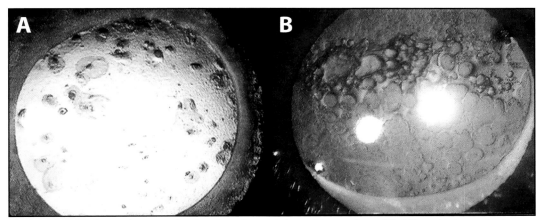

Figure 14-5. Slit-lamp photographs showing pigment deposition surface of 2 different intraocular lenses. This complication is not uncommon after the pediatric cataract surgery and usually does not cause a decrease in visual acuity. (Reprinted with permission from Pandey SK, Wilson E. Principles and paradigms of pediatric cataract surgery and intraocular lens implantation. In: Agarwal A, ed. *Phaco Nightmares: Conquering Cataract Catastrophes*. Thorofare, NJ: SLACK Incorporated; 2006:65-98.)

Summary

Microbimanual techniques (or microphakonit) represent a nice improvement in the management of cataracts in the adult, and some of its main advantages can be used to solve some of the technical troubles that we frequently find in the pediatric cataract. We believe that it is a good option because it is minimally invasive, provides access to all meridians, offers an improvement in fluidics management, and increases the safety of some maneuvers; for example, the management of the posterior capsule and bi-axial vitrectomy is feasible through the same incisions.

References

1. Vejarano LF, Tello A, Vejarano A. Phakonit: incisions and use of a pressurized inflow system. *J Cataract Refract Surg*. 2004;30(5):939.
2. Agarwal A, Agarwal S, Agarwal A. Phakonit and laser phakonit: lens removal through a 0.9-mm incision. In: Agarwal A, Agarwal S, Agarwal A, eds. *Phacoemulsification, Laser Cataract Surgery and Foldable IOL's*. 2nd ed. New Delhi, India: Jaypee; 2000:204-216.
3. Agarwal A. *Bimanual Phaco. Mastering the Phakonit/MICS Technique*. Thorofare, NJ: SLACK Incorporated; 2004.
4. Seibel BS. Physics of capsulorhexis. In: Seibel BS, ed. *Phacodynamics*. New York, NY: McGraw-Hill; 1993:146-147.
5. Gimbel HV, DeBroff BM. Posterior capsulorhexis with optic capture: maintaining a clear visual axis after pediatric cataract surgery. *J Cataract Refract Surgery*. 1994;20(6):658-664.
6. Wilson ME, Bluestein EC, Wang XH, Apple DJ. Comparison of mechanized anterior capsulectomy and manual continuous capsulorhexis in pediatric eyes. *J Cataract Refract Surg*. 1994;20(6):602-606.
7. Pèrez-Arteaga A. Management of pediatric cataract extraction with 700 micron technology for lens removal. Paper presented at: ASCRS Meeting; 2008; Chicago.
8. Pèrez-Arteaga A. Transoperative IOL power calculation. In: Ashok G, ed. *Mastering the Techniques of IOL Power Calculations*. New Delhi, India: Jaypee Brothers; 2008.
9. Pérez-Arteaga A. Anterior vented gas forced infusion of the Accurus Surgical System for phakonit. *J Cataract Refract Surg*. 2004; 30(4):933-935.
10. Agarwal A. Microphakonit surgery performed with 0.7-mm tip. *Ocul Surg News. Eur. Asia Pac. Ed*. September 2005.

CHAPTER 15

MICROINCISIONAL CATARACT SURGERY COMBINED WITH OTHER SURGERIES

Archana Nair, MS; Dhivya Ashok Kumar, MD; and Amar Agarwal, MS, FRCS, FRCOphth

Cataract surgery in combination with other surgical interventions for coexisting ocular conditions like glaucoma and corneal or retinal disorders has been in practice for a long time. Earlier cataract extraction was performed alone, followed by cataract removal with intraocular lens (IOL) implantation.[1,2] Later on, cataract surgeries were combined with penetrating keratoplasty (triple procedure), glaucoma surgeries (trabeculectomy), and posterior segment interventions (pars plana vitrectomy).[3,4] Subsequently, after the invention of phacoemulsification, the surgical space for combining other procedures in the same sitting has increased.[5-7] Thus, these combination techniques, with their ability to give good functional results equivalent to isolated procedures, have reduced the need for repeat surgeries. Microincisional cataract surgeries (MICS) can also be combined with other procedures within the same sitting similar to conventional phacoemulsification. Microincisional surgeries,[8-11] namely microphakonit (700-μm) or phakonit (900-μm), along with other procedures can be done with rapidity and minimal trauma to the eye.

700-MICRON CATARACT SURGERY WITH TRANSCLERAL 20-GAUGE PARS PLANA VITRECTOMY

Clear corneal incision with an Agarwal 800-μm microphakonit knife (MicroSurgical Technology, Redmond, WA) is made initially for the main port and the side port, and capsulorrhexis is done. Capsulorrhexis is followed by gentle hydrodissection and nucleus rotation. The nucleus is emulsified with a 700-μm sleeveless phaco needle (MicroSurgical Technology) connected to an aspiration line and irrigating chopper connected to the infusion line of the phaco machine. A 700-μm bimanual irrigation/aspiration set (MicroSurgical Technology) is used for cortical aspiration. Gas-forced infusion with an air pump is used during the entire procedure.[12] The clear corneal wound is hydrated without sutures. An infusion cannula is inserted in the pars plana about 3.5 mm from the limbus and 2 additional pars plana sclerotomies are made. Pars plana vitrectomy is performed safely (Figure 15-1). Sclerotomy wounds are closed with polyglactin suture. The conjunctiva is also closed with sutures.

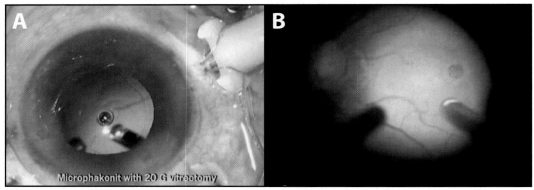

Figure 15-1. (A) Pars plana vitrectomy performed after cataract removal with microphakonit. (B) Fundus view as seen with the wide angle in pars plana vitrectomy after microphakonit.

700-MICRON CATARACT SURGERY WITH 25-GAUGE TRANSCONJUNCTIVAL SUTURELESS VITRECTOMY

Cataract removal is done in the standard way with 700-μm instruments. At the end of surgery, the stromal wound hydration is done. An initial transconjunctival 25-gauge vitrectomy trocar is inserted in the inferotemporal quadrant. Two additional transconjunctival 25-gauge trocars are also inserted (Figure 15-2A). A 25-gauge cannula connected to an infusion line is then inserted in the inferotemporal quadrant (Figure 15-2B). Transconjunctival pars plana vitrectomy is performed.[13] The cataract wounds are small, stable (Figure 15-3), self-sealing,[14] and able to withstand high intravitreal pressures during vitrectomy without leakage, chamber shallowing, or iris prolapse. The problem of reduced globe resistance and wound instability during infusion cannula insertion is not encountered with this technique. Therefore, unlike the earlier transconjunctival sutureless vitrectomy technique in which the infusion cannula is inserted before phacoemulsification, here the infusion cannula can be inserted after cataract extraction with 700-μm instruments. The main-port cataract incision also does not have to be sutured, unlike in conventionally performed combined coaxial phacoemulsification with vitrectomy. Thus, this combination of microphakonit with transconjunctival vitrectomy makes the combined procedure more rapid and minimally invasive.

700-MICRON CATARACT SURGERY WITH GLUED 20-GAUGE SUTURELESS VITRECTOMY

Microphakonit with 700-μm instruments is used to remove cataract followed by 20-gauge sutureless vitrectomy. Vitreous hemorrhages with cataract or vitreous membranes with cataract extraction are the common indications. Three partial-thickness scleral flaps are made (Figure 15-4). The first flap (F1) is made in the inferotemporal quadrant. The next 2 flaps (F2, F3) are made in the superior nasal and superior temporal quadrants about 2 mm from the limbus. A straight sclerotomy is made under the scleral flap F1 about 3.5 mm from the limbus. A polyglactin 6-0 suture is placed and a 4-mm infusion cannula connected to a 500-mL bottle of balanced salt solution is inserted through the sclerotomy. Two straight sclerotomies with a 20-gauge needle are made under the existing scleral flaps (F1, F2). Pars plana vitrectomy is completed with 20-gauge vitrectomy instruments (vitrectomy probe and endoilluminator).

MICROINCISIONAL CATARACT SURGERY COMBINED WITH OTHER SURGERIES

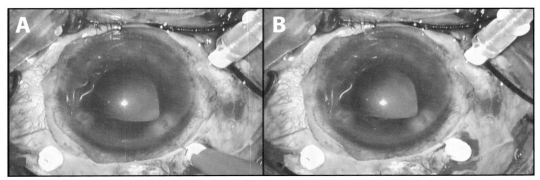

Figure 15-2. (A) 25-gauge pars plana transconjunctival trocar inserted after 700-μm cataract surgery. (B) 25-gauge transconjunctival to be started.

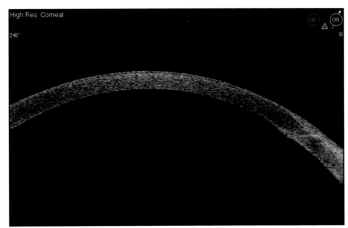

Figure 15-3. Anterior segment optical coherence tomography picture showing the self-sealed 700-μm clear corneal wound.

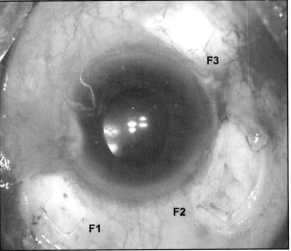

Figure 15-4. Intraoperative photograph showing the 3 partial-thickness scleral flaps (F1, F2, F3) being made for glued 20-gauge sutureless vitrectomy.

At the end of the procedure, the polyglactin suture and the infusion cannula are removed and the scleral flaps (F1, F2, F3) are sealed with the tissue glue (Tisseel, Baxter, Deerfield, IL). The conjunctiva is also apposed at the peritomy sites with the glue.

700-Micron Cataract Surgery With Trabeculectomy

In eyes with coexisting cataract with glaucoma, MICS can be combined with trabeculectomy. In this procedure, an initial superior limbal partial-thickness scleral flap is made for trabeculectomy. Then, the clear corneal incisions with an 800-µm microphakonit knife are made for the main port and the side port and capsulorrhexis is done. Cataract is removed with 700-µm instruments and a foldable IOL is implanted after extension of the wound. Trabeculectomy is performed under the existing scleral flap (Figure 15-5), followed by peripheral iridectomy. The scleral flap is sutured followed by conjunctival closure.

700-Micron Cataract Surgery in No-Anesthesia Cataract Surgery

Combinations of 700-µm cataract surgery with no anesthesia can be done.[15-17] The incisions used for microphakonit are so small and self-sealing that the chances of them opening up due to lid or ocular movements is negligible. This makes the entry of periocular bacteria into the eye postoperatively a remote possibility. Moreover, a topical anesthetic agent and its vehicle may serve as a reservoir of microbial contamination with the potential to cause infection. Other disadvantages with topical anesthesia include possible corneal epithelial, corneal endothelial, or retinal toxicity, which is mainly the result of the preservatives in the anesthetic solutions. Some agents (eg, proparacaine) can also lead to allergic and idiosyncratic reactions such as periocular swelling, erythema, and contact dermatitis. In addition, preoperative instillation of some topical anesthetic agents (eg, lidocaine) can cause burning and stinging, and multiple applications can lead to mild corneal haziness during surgery. Use of intracameral preservative-free xylocaine may cause endothelial toxicity. These combination techniques of microphakonit with no anesthesia will help in combating postoperative endophthalmitis—one of the most dreaded and devastating complications of cataract surgery.

Microincisional Cataract Surgery Combined With Other Procedures

MICS can be combined with iris retracting hooks (Figure 15-6) in eyes with small pupils or with endocapsular ring implantation (Figure 15-7) in eyes with subluxated cataract. Other simple procedures like intravitreal injections of anti-vascular endothelial growth factor or steroid injection can also be combined.

Advantages of Microincisional Cataract Surgery Combined Surgeries

According to Park et al, combined phacoemulsification and pars plana vitrectomy (23- and 20-gauge) can induce significant surgical-induced astigmatism at postoperative week 1 and decrease over 3 months.[18] It has also been shown that combined surgeries do not induce significant astigmatic change per se, and the astigmatism will be the same when either procedure is performed alone.[19] Nevertheless, microphakonit with pars plana vitrectomy has less chance of induced astigmatism due to its small incision size and absence of sutures. This also reduces the suture-related clear corneal infections as reported previously.[20] Operative complications like wound leakage, chamber shallowing, or iris prolapse can also be minimized. Combination techniques of microphakonit will also help in reducing the incidence of postoperative endophthalmitis.[17]

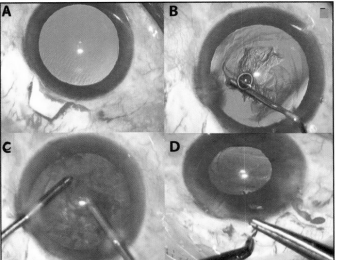

Figure 15-5. (A) Superior partial-thickness scleral flap made for combined surgery of cataract and glaucoma. (B) Intraoperative image showing the hydrodissection being done. (C) 700-µm phaco needle and irrigating chopper used for cataract removal. (D) Trabeculectomy is performed and scleral flap closed with sutures.

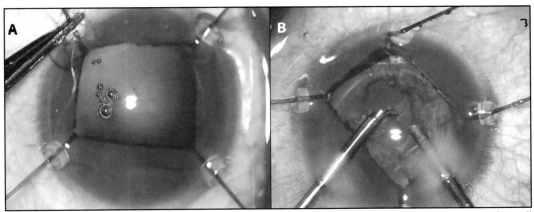

Figure 15-6. (A) Intraoperative picture showing the use of iris retracting hooks in MICS in eyes with small pupils. (B) Microphakonit is performed.

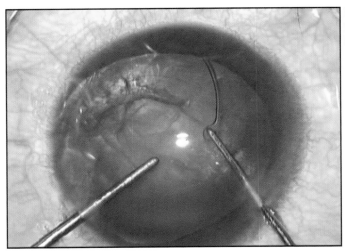

Figure 15-7. Endocapsular ring is inserted in a subluxated cataract before doing microphakonit.

Summary

With the advantage of microincisional surgeries, it is possible to do combined procedures rapidly and with minimal trauma. We believe that these combination techniques along with developments in IOL technology such as smaller IOLs or injectable IOLs may significantly improve surgical results in the near future. There is no doubt that the development of MICS has improved the success rate and reduced the complication rate previously associated with large-incision combined techniques.

References

1. Agarwal A. *Phaco Nightmares: Conquering Cataract Catastrophes*. Thorofare, NJ: SLACK Incorporated; 2006.
2. Agarwal S, Agarwal A, Agarwal A. *Phacoemulsification*. 3rd ed. Delhi, India: Jaypee Brothers; 2004.
3. McCartney DL, Memmen JE, Stark WJ, et al. The efficacy and safety of combined trabeculectomy, cataract extraction, and intraocular lens implantation. *Ophthalmology*. 1988;95(6):754-762.
4. Green M, Chow A, Apel A. Outcomes of combined penetrating keratoplasty and cataract extraction compared with penetrating keratoplasty alone. *Clin Experiment Ophthalmol*. 2007;35(4):324-329.
5. Tham CC, Kwong YY, Leung DY, et al. Phacoemulsification versus combined phacotrabeculectomy in medically uncontrolled chronic angle closure glaucoma with cataracts. *Ophthalmology*. 2009;116(4):725-731.
6. Terry MA, Shamie N, Chen ES, et al. Endothelial keratoplasty for Fuchs' dystrophy with cataract: complications and clinical results with the new triple procedure. *Ophthalmology*. 2009;116(4):631-639.
7. Hwang JU, Yoon YH, Kim DS, Kim JG. Combined phacoemulsification, foldable intraocular lens implantation, and 25-gauge transconjunctival sutureless vitrectomy. *J Cataract Refract Surg*. 2006;32(5):727-731.
8. Pandey SK, Werner L, Agarwal A, et al. Phakonit: cataract removal through a sub-1.0 mm incision with implantation of the ThinOptX rollable intraocular lens. *J Cataract Refract Surg*. 2002;28(9):1710-1713.
9. Agarwal A, Agarwal A, Agarwal S, Narang P, Narang S. Phakonit: phacoemulsification through a 0.9 mm corneal incision. *J Cataract Refract Surg*. 2001;27:1548-1552.
10. Agarwal A, Agarwal S, Agarwal A. Phakonit with an AcriTec IOL. *J Cataract Refract Surg*. 2003;29(4):854-855.
11. Agarwal A, Trivedi RH, Jacob S, Agarwal A, Agarwal S. Microphakonit: 700 micron cataract surgery. *Clin Ophthalmol*. 2007;1(3):323-325.
12. Agarwal A, Agarwal S, Agarwal A, Lal V, Patel N. Antichamber collapser. *J Cataract Refract Surg*. 2002;28(7):1085-1086.
13. Agarwal A, Jacob S, Agarwal A. Combined microphakonit and 25-gauge transconjunctival sutureless vitrectomy. *J Cataract Refract Surg*. 2007;33(11):1839-1840.
14. Agarwal A, Kumar DA, Jacob S, Agarwal A. In vivo analysis of wound architecture in 700 microm microphakonit cataract surgery. *J Cataract Refract Surg*. 2008;34(9):1554-1560.
15. Suresh K, Pandey L, Werner DJ, et al. No anaesthesia clear corneal phacoemulsification versus topical and topical plus intracameral anaesthesia: randomized clinical trial. *J Cataract Refract Surg*. 2001;27(10):1643-1650.
16. Rosenwasser GO. Complications of topical ocular anesthetics. *Int Ophthalmol Clin*. 1989;29(3):153-158.
17. Agarwal A, Jacob S, Sinha S, Agarwal A. Combating endophthalmitis with microphakonit and no-anesthesia technique. *J Cataract Refract Surg*. 2007;33(12):2009-2011.
18. Park DH, Shin JP, Kim SY. Surgically induced astigmatism in combined phacoemulsification and vitrectomy; 23-gauge transconjunctival sutureless vitrectomy versus 20-gauge standard vitrectomy. *Graefe's Arch Clin Exp Ophthalmol*. 2009;247(10):1331-1337.
19. Yuen YF, Cheung TOB, Tsang CW, Lam RF, Baig NB, Lam SCD. Surgically induced astigmatism in phacoemulsification, pars plana vitrectomy, and combined phacoemulsification and vitrectomy: a comparative study. *Eye*. 2009;23(3):576-580.
20. Lee BJ, Smith SD, Jeng BH. Suture-related corneal infections after clear corneal cataract surgery. *J Cataract Refract Surg*. 2009;35(5):939-942.

SECTION IV
MICROINCISIONAL LENSES AND COMPLICATION MANAGEMENT

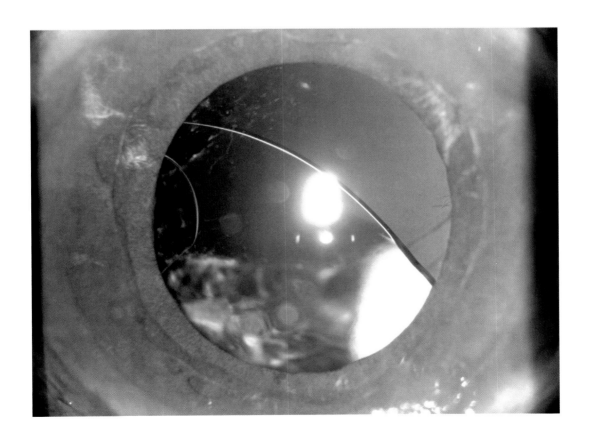

CHAPTER 16

MICS Injector Systems

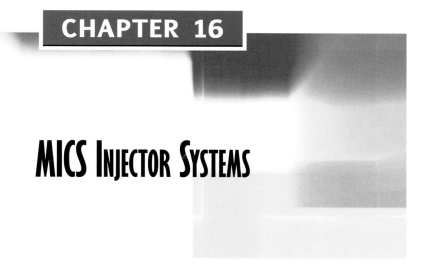

Kelly J. Grimes, MS and Bonnie An Henderson, MD

Microincisional cataract surgery (MICS) is not complete unless implantation of an intraocular lens (IOL) can be achieved through the same small incision. The success of delivering an IOL through a microincision is dependent on 2 factors: the ability of the IOL to be compressed sufficiently to pass through the small incision and the ability to create a delivery system for the IOL that will also pass through the same small incision. Originally, foldable IOLs were manually folded and placed into the eye with a forceps. Implantation of foldable IOLs has evolved over the past 2 decades to include IOL injector systems.

INJECTOR SYSTEMS

Injector systems are used during phacoemulsification cataract surgery to inject the IOL into the capsular bag through a narrow tube placed within the corneal incision. The main goal of using an injector system is to allow the implantation of a normal-sized IOL through a much smaller microincision. Injector systems include a cartridge where the lens is held until delivery into the eye. The use of cartridges and injector systems minimizes the use of forceps, which can scratch the lens and cause spherical aberrations.[1] Injector systems allow the surgeon to introduce the lens into the eye without the lens actually touching the incision or the conjunctiva. This offers a certain sterile advantage over previous techniques, which relied on the use of forceps to place the lens into the eye.

TWISTING AND PLUNGER METHOD

A variety of injector systems are currently available. Injector systems vary in dimension and material. Therefore, it is important to match an IOL with a compatible injector system because injectors can only be used with certain IOLs. Injectors push the lens forward into the eye via 2 mechanisms. The micrometer advance (twist) mechanism involves a bimanual screw-like motion where the surgeon rotates the upper portion of the injector, slowly pushing the IOL forward into the capsular bag. In the syringe advance (plunger) mechanism, the physician simply pushes the IOL forward using a plunger-style motion.

Several attributes are associated with both mechanisms that should be considered when choosing between the 2. Although the plunger method is more intuitive, the twist method allows the surgeon to halt the advancement of the lens if repositioning is required. Furthermore, the micrometer advance allows for finer control over injection power. The plunger method allows the surgeon to only use one hand, freeing the other to stabilize the eye in an uncooperative patient. The plunger method also allows for greater feedback because the surgeon can better sense resistance during lens injection.

PRELOADED INJECTORS

Preloaded injectors come loaded with the patient's appropriate lens, thus removing the need to load each injector with a lens prior to surgery. This provides 3 main advantages. First, preloaded injectors can decrease the chance of human error because the nursing staff does not have to load the patient-specific lens immediately prior to surgery. Second, preloaded injectors can lower the chance of creating iatrogenic aberrations on the lens during loading. Most importantly, preloaded injectors can improve sterility and decrease the chance of contamination because the lens is never manipulated after production.

Currently, preloaded lenses are being used in Europe and Japan. Commercially available lenses include Hoya 2.3-mm incision (Chino Hills, CA), Carl Zeiss Meditec AG 2.8 mm (Jena, Germany), STAAR 2.75 mm (Monrovia, CA), Hoya iSert, and Quatrix Aspheric Preloaded 2.8 mm (Croma-Pharma, Leobendorf, Austria). Alcon (Fort Worth, TX) is planning to introduce the AcrySert C in the United States, allowing surgeons to take advantage of this emerging technology.

MONARCH III WITH D CARTRIDGE

The Monarch III D cartridge (Alcon) offers a 2.2-mm incision injection system for use with all AcrySof IOLs (Alcon; Figure 16-1). Despite allowing the surgeon to operate through a smaller incision, the D cartridge actually offers a larger loading dock (6.0 mm) from its predecessor, the C cartridge (5.5 mm).[2] This allows for easier loading without sacrificing an increase in incision size. The smaller D cartridge allows for an easier delivery of the lens with little to no enlargement of the corneal incision after lens delivery. The Monarch III requires the lens to be loaded with forceps prior to injection. Before loading the lens, a dispersive viscoelastic is introduced into the cartridge loading chamber. The IOL is then placed into the chamber with both haptics folded onto the anterior surface of the optic. The cartridge is then loaded into the injector. The injector tip enters the 2.2-mm incision bevel down and, using a continuous twisting motion, the IOL is introduced into the anterior chamber. The DK7797-2 (Duckworth & Kent, Hertfordshire, UK) and the Royale II Unihand Spring Injector (ASICO, Westmont, IL) are also compatible with the C cartridge and AcrySof IOLs.

STAAR NANOPOINT

The Nanopoint (STAAR, Monrovia, CA) is a plunger-style, single-use injector that allows lens injection through a 2.2-mm incision (Figure 16-2). The Nanopoint is to be used with the STAAR Afinity Collamer Single-Piece IOL.[3] A loading block is used to load the IOL into the provided cartridge. Some surgeons may find the Collamer IOLs to be flexible and easier to fit through a microincision and into the anterior chamber.

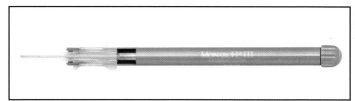

Figure 16-1. Monarch III D cartridge. (Reprinted with permission from Alcon, Fort Worth, TX.)

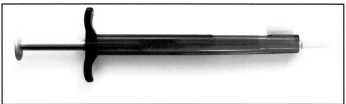

Figure 16-2. Nanopoint injector. (Reprinted with permission from STAAR, Monrovia, CA.)

MicroSTAAR Injectors

STAAR offers 3 other injectors, with both plunger and twist advance mechanisms for 2.8-mm incisions. All MicroSTAAR injectors are compatible with the AQ Cartridge (to be used with STAAR Elastimide Lens [3-piece silicone IOL], which has 45-degree beveled edge with 2 slits) or an MTC-60c cartridge (to be used with STAAR Elastic Lens [single-piece silicone IOL] with a 60-degree beveled edge and no slits). The MicroSTAAR injectors are autoclavable and meant for multiple uses.

STAAR Preloaded Intraocular Lens

The STAAR Preloaded IOL system removes the loading step, improving sterility and efficiency. The model KS-3Ai IOL comes preloaded in an injector with the option for a push or twist injection action.

ThinOptX Rollable Intraocular Lens

The ThinOptX Ultrachoice 1.0 lens (Abingdon, VA) and injector system allows injection of an IOL through an unenlarged 1.5-mm incision.[4-10] Currently, ThinOptX provides an injector system (Figure 16-3) that allows for the smallest incision sizes currently used in practice. The lens is not preloaded and must be rolled into the injector prior to delivery.

With the availability of the ThinOptX rollable IOL, which can be inserted through sub-1.5-mm incision, the full potential of phakonit can be realized. This lens was created and designed by Wayne Callahan from the United States. The first such ultrathin lens was implanted by Jairo Hoyos from Spain. Subsequently, on October 2, 2001, Amar Agarwal modified the lens by making the optic size 5 mm so that it could go through a smaller incision (Figure 16-4).

Unfolder Emerald Series

The Unfolder Emerald Series injector system (Figure 16-5) offered by Abbott Medical Optics (Santa Ana, CA) is designed for use with their acrylic IOLs, including the ReZoom multifocal IOL, TECNIS acrylic ashperic monofocal and multifocal IOLs, and the Sensar IOL.

Figure 16-3. ThinOptX roller cum injector inserting the IOL in the capsular bag.[11] (Photo courtesy of Dr. Agarwal's Group of Eye Hospitals and Eye Research Centre, Chennai, India.)

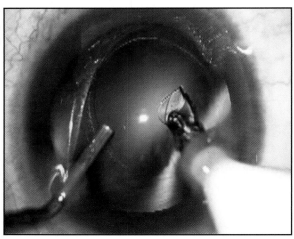

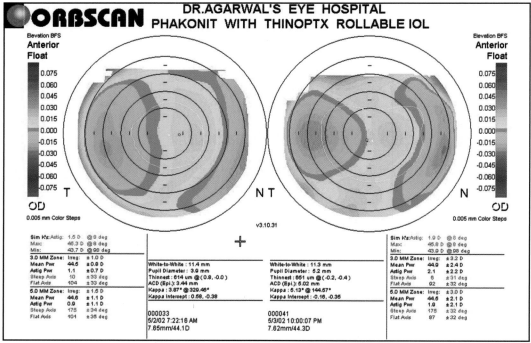

Figure 16-4. Topograpy with the ThinOptX rollable IOL after phakonit.[11] (Photo courtesy of Dr. Agarwal's Group of Eye Hospitals and Eye Research Centre, Chennai, India.)

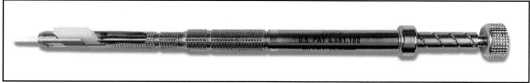

Figure 16-5. Unfolder Emerald Series injector system. (Reprinted with permission from Abbott Medical Optics, Santa Ana, CA.)

The injector can be used with a 2.6-mm incision. To load the IOL into the cartridge, begin by opening the cartridge so that the cartridge tray opens surface side up (upright) into the sterile field. Like most injector systems, the Unfolder series injectors require viscoelastic to be loaded into the cartridge chamber prior to IOL loading. Load a cohesive viscoelastic into the chamber of the cartridge, where the lens will travel through in the final steps of injection. Apply a line of viscoelastic on the upper and lower troughs of the chamber. Place a single drop of viscoelastic on the loading dock. Using forceps, place the IOL onto the loading dock and gently slide it into the chamber. The IOL should be loaded in a similar orientation as illustrated by the IOL outline printed on the chamber wing. Once the IOL is slid into the chamber, make sure that the IOL is below the ledges of the chamber. Close the cartridge, ensuring that the leading haptic is facing forward and the trailing haptic is exiting out the back of the cartridge. Load the cartridge into the slot on the injector handpiece. Slide the cartridge forward so that the cartridge tube extends fully forward out of the handpiece opening. The Unfolder series has a 2-step process for advancing the lens through the injector chamber and into the eye. Before entering the eye, push the plunger forward until the marked screw pattern on the plunger shaft enters the handpiece body. Advance the lens further by twisting using the screw mechanisms until the IOL is visible in the cartridge tube. Enter the eye via a 2.6-mm incision and introduce the IOL into the capsular bag using the twist mechanism.

UNFOLDER SILVER SERIES

Abbott Medical Optics offers the Unfolder Silver Series (Figure 16-6) for use with their silicone IOLs (PhacoFlex II, SI40, ClariFlex, CeeOn, and Technis IOLs). Like the Emerald Series, the Silver Series requires a technician to load the lens onto a cartridge that attaches the latter to the inserter. To begin, the cartridge lid is opened. Using the provided Unfolder Silver handpiece, load a cohesive viscoelastic onto the upper and lower troughs, backfill the barrel of the cartridge, and apply one drop of a cohesive viscoelastic onto the middle of the cartridge trough. Be sure not to overfill the chamber with viscoelastic because silicone IOLs require less in the loading cartridge than do acrylic IOLs. To load the IOL into the cartridge, make sure the leading haptic is facing forward in the barrel and use a forceps to push down on the outer edge of the optic to push the IOL under the ledges of the cartridge chamber. The trailing haptic should exit the chamber and there should be no viscoelastic on the upper face of the IOL. Secure the IOL into the chamber by closing the wings and snapping them shut. The cartridge is now ready to be inserted into the handpiece. The Unfolder Silver Series requires a 2.8-mm incision for insertion of the IOL into the capsular bag. Use the plunger mechanism to push the IOL forward to the tip of the injector. Place the injector tip into the 2.8-mm incision and use the twist mechanism to introduce the IOL into the capsular bag.

SOFPORT INJECTOR SYSTEM

The Easy-Load Inserter of the SofPort Injector System (Bausch & Lomb, Aliso Viejo, CA) is a single-use, syringe-shaped injector designed to be used with the LI61AO 3-piece IOL. The Easy-Load Inserter injects the lens into the eye through a sub-3-mm incision with minimal manipulation of the lens. The IOL comes in a lens case that attaches directly to the cartridge, allowing the technician to load the lens without actually touching the lens, helping to maintain sterility. The body tip is protected by a haptic cover that is removed in the final step prior to injection. The Easy-Load Inserter offers a transparent cartridge and tip, allowing the surgeon to visualize the lens as it moves from the cartridge, through the

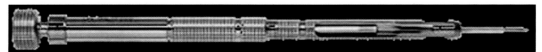

Figure 16-6. Unfolder Silver Series injector system. (Reprinted with permission from Abbott Medical Optics, Santa Ana, CA.)

body tip, and into the capsular bag. A special feature of the SofPort injector system is the M-fold lens, which introduces the lens into the capsular bag in a flat, plantar orientation, minimizing the need for lens readjustment.

HOYA GREEN SERIES

The Hoya Green Series IS is a reusable injection system designed for MICS. The Green Series IS utilizes the F-18 cartridge system, which must first be loaded with viscoelastic prior to loading the lens. Next, remove the IOL from the IOL case and load it into the cartridge, ensuring that the leading haptic is extending forward as illustrated by the haptic mark on the cartridge. To implant, insert the cartridge into the incision, turning the tip of the cartridge upward. As the IOL is introduced, the leading haptic should extend to the left. Slowly rotate the handpiece 270 degrees to the left—this motion should introduce the optic and the trailing haptic into the capsular bag.

HOYA ISERT PRELOADED INJECTOR

Hoya offers a preloaded MICS injector system that is currently only available outside of the United States. The iSert injector is a disposable, single-use injector eliminating the need for sterilization while potentially reducing loading errors. To begin, load low- to medium-viscosity viscoelastic (avoid using highly viscous viscoelastics) through the opening until the viscoelastic reaches the cover case. Next, detach the cover case and slowly push the plunger forward to advance the IOL, making sure that the leading haptic begins to extend. Continue to push the plunger forward and stop once it cannot be advanced any longer. The surgeon may need to rotate the plunger to advance the IOL to the bevel tip immediately prior to implanting the IOL into the eye. To implant the IOL, enter the eye bevel down, continuously twisting the plunger to the right. The leading haptic should extend to the left as the IOL begins to enter the eye. Once the leading haptic is below the capsulorrhexis, rotate the injector counterclockwise. This motion should force the IOL out of the injector with the folded portion of the IOL facing the posterior capsule. Continue to rotate the injector until the entire IOL is implanted into the eye.

SUMMARY

As incision sizes for cataract surgery continue to decrease, new microincision-compatible IOLs are constantly being created worldwide. With the introduction of these new and thinner IOLs, the injector systems also continue to evolve to allow the surgeon to place IOLs through increasingly smaller incision sizes. These injector systems have greatly improved the safety of MICS while consistently delivering an undamaged IOL.

REFERENCES

1. Gunenc U, Oner FH, Tongal S, Ferliel M. Effects on visual function of glistenings and folding marks in Acry-Sof intraocular lenses. *J Cataract Refract Surg.* 2001;27(10):1611-1614.
2. Tkia KF. Advances in microcoaxial phaco: near-future product launches for the Intrepid system. *Cataract Refract Surg Today Eur.* 2007;21-22.
3. Sanders DR, Doney K, Poco M, ICL in Treatment of Myopia Study Group. United States Food and Drug Administration clinical trial of the implantable Collamer lens (ICL) for moderate to high myopia. *Ophthalmology.* 2004;111(9):1683-1692.
4. Agarwal A, Agarwal A, Agarwal S, Narang P, Narang S. Phakonit: phacoemulsification through a 0.9 mm corneal incision. *J Cataract Refract Surg.* 2001;27(10):1548-1552.
5. Agarwal A, Agarwal S, Agarwal A. Phakonit with an AcriTec IOL. *Ophthalmology.* 2003;29(4):854-855.
6. Pandey SK, Wener L, Agarwal A, et al. Phakonit: Cataract removal through a sub 1.0 mm incision with implantation of the ThinOptX rollable IOL. *J Cataract Refract Surg.* 2002;28(9):1710-1713.
7. Agarwal A, Trivedi RH, Jacob S, Agarwal A, Agarwal S. Microphakonit: 700 micron cataract surgery. *Clin Ophthalmol.* 2007;1(3):323-325.
8. Agarwal A, Jacob S, Agarwal A. Combined microphakonit and 25-gauge transconjunctival sutureless vitrectomy. *J Cataract Refract Surg.* 2007;33(11):1839-1840.
9. Agarwal A, Jacob S, Sinha S, Agarwal A. Combating endophthalmitis with microphakonit and no-anesthesia technique. *J Cataract Refract Surg.* 2008;33(12):2009-2011.
10. Agarwal A, Kumar DA, Jacob S, Agarwal A. In vivo analysis of wound architecture in 700 micron microphakonit surgery. *J Cataract Refract Surg.* 2008;34(9):1554-1560.
11. Agarwal A. *Bimanual Phaco: Mastering the Phakonit/MICS Technique.* Thorofare, NJ: SLACK Incorporated; 2004.

CHAPTER 17

MICROINCISIONAL INTRAOCULAR LENSES

*Mayank A. Nanavaty, DO, MRCOphth, MRCS(Ed)
and David J. Spalton, FRCP, FRCS, FRCOphth*

Cataract surgery has undergone remarkable changes in recent decades with the development of phacoemulsification in the late 1960s and foldable intraocular lenses (IOLs) in the late 1980s. These continuing developments have made microincisional cataract surgery (MICS) possible. Incision size has dropped from 3.0 mm or more to 1.5 mm or less, and even some coaxial phacoemulsification equipment can now be used through surgical wounds closer to 2.0 mm rather than 3.0 mm. As incision size decreases, so does the rehabilitation time, along with reduced chances of complications such as induced astigmatism and endophthalmitis. Microincision can be defined as sub-2.0-mm incision size, usually requiring a bimanual phacoemulsification technique. To take advantage of the reduced incision size, thin, flexible IOLs that can be inserted through a sub-2.0-mm opening are required. In theory, ultrathin lenses have the advantage of insertion through smaller incisions and they are potentially more optically perfect because optical aberrations increase with lens thickness.

FOLDABLE INTRAOCULAR LENSES

Standard single-piece hydrophobic and hydrophilic acrylic IOLs designed for 3-mm incisions, with some adaptation, may be implanted through smaller incisions by using a cartridge with a smaller tip and by using wound-assisted implantation, but generally microincisional lenses are inserted using a wound-assisted technique in a purpose-designed cartridge lubricated with viscoelastic and protected from damage during insertion by a silicone pad on the piston. The Akreos Adapt (Figure 17-1; Bausch & Lomb, Aliso Viejo, CA), the AcrySof SA60 series (Alcon, Fort Worth, TX), and the Xcelens Idea (Croma-Pharma, Leobendorf, Austria) are a few examples of IOLs for which this approach can be used. In addition, aspheric designs and the high refractive index of some IOL materials allow a thinner optic, thus reducing the thickness of the IOL when folded. The advantage of this approach lies in the ability to implant standard high-quality IOLs through smaller incisions. The disadvantage is that none of these IOLs can be safely implanted through incisions of 2 mm or less throughout the whole dioptric range.

CHAPTER 17

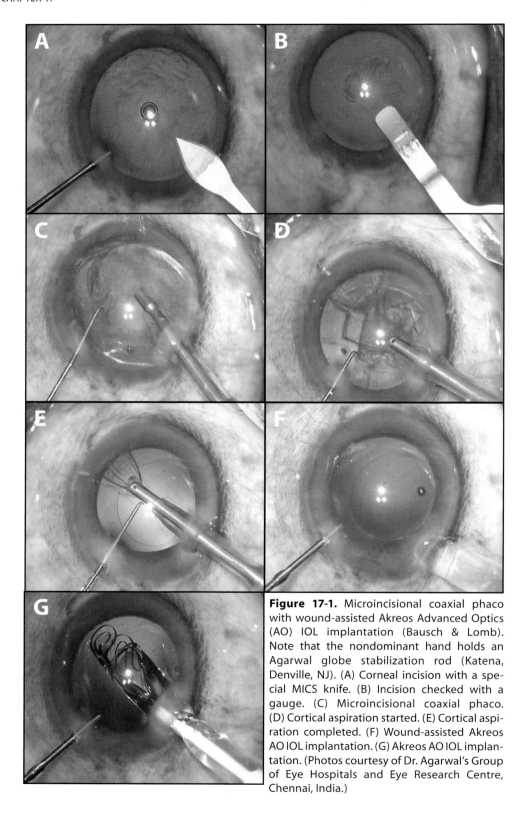

Figure 17-1. Microincisional coaxial phaco with wound-assisted Akreos Advanced Optics (AO) IOL implantation (Bausch & Lomb). Note that the nondominant hand holds an Agarwal globe stabilization rod (Katena, Denville, NJ). (A) Corneal incision with a special MICS knife. (B) Incision checked with a gauge. (C) Microincisional coaxial phaco. (D) Cortical aspiration started. (E) Cortical aspiration completed. (F) Wound-assisted Akreos AO IOL implantation. (G) Akreos AO IOL implantation. (Photos courtesy of Dr. Agarwal's Group of Eye Hospitals and Eye Research Centre, Chennai, India.)

MICROINCISIONAL INTRAOCULAR LENSES

True microincisional surgery necessitates smaller and thinner IOL designs that can be implanted through sub-2-mm incisions; such IOLs cannot simply be smaller versions of a larger IOL. The introduction of the Ultrachoice 1.0 lens (ThinOptX, Abingdon, VA) opened the discussion on how to manufacture the IOL to reach the incision size objective without compromising on optical quality (Figure 17-2). This IOL had a thickness of 350 μm and an optic that was a combination of peripheral Fresnel lenses with a central traditional spherical optic. It was rolled for insertion. It suffered from the problems of dysphotopic symptoms from the Fresnel element and buckling from capsular contraction. The Acri.Tec Acri.Smart IOL (Carl Zeiss Meditec, Jena, Germany) has obtained wide acceptance in Europe. More recently, other microincisional IOLs with different designs have been introduced (eg, HumanOptics, Erlangen, Germany; Bausch & Lomb) and the impression is that we are facing a further evolution of cataract surgery.

Developing microincisional lenses has been fraught with technical challenges. They must be soft and flexible enough to fold into a small cartridge, yet sturdy enough to resist tearing during insertion and thin enough to fold up while retaining sufficient refractive power for a wide range of IOL powers, in addition to offering optical performance and resistance to decentration from capsular fibrosis and posterior capsular opacification comparable to existing standard lenses. Though these challenges are substantial, many companies have now started manufacturing them. As a result, a range of lenses are now available that can be inserted through a 2.2-mm down to a 1.5-mm microincision level.

ACRI.TEC INTRAOCULAR LENSES

Founded in 1997 by Dr. Christine Kreiner, Acri.Tec (now part of Zeiss) was one of the first manufacturers to develop a microincisional lens. The rollable Acri.Smart lens was first implanted through a 2.0-mm incision in 2000 and was on the market in Europe in December 2001. The company, based in Heningsdorf, Germany, now offers a wide range of lenses based on the original Acri.Smart design, including spheric, aspheric, neutrally aspheric, toric, multifocal, and multifocal toric versions in powers from 0 to +32 diopters. The design of the Acri.Smart IOL series is simple: it is a one-piece, plate-haptic, foldable acrylic IOL with a water content of 25% and with hydrophobic surfaces (Table 17-1). These lenses can be considered to be an evolution from older silicone models, with the acrylic material favoring better and more stable fixation. The refractive index is 1.46, the central thickness is approximately 0.7 mm, the edge thickness is 0.25 to 0.27 mm, and the diameter of a 19.00 D rolled lens is 1.3 mm.[1] The lens can be implanted through a sub-2-mm incision. Because of its efficacy and success, several modifications were implemented with the purpose of meeting specific needs: the toric model (Acri.Comfort 646 TLC) and the multifocal (Acri.LISA 366D). Most recently, a combination of these 2 variations has been launched: the Acri.LISA Toric 466TD. This lens has a toric anterior surface and a diffractive design 3.75 D add on the posterior surface, providing a 2:1 ratio of light focused to distance and near. Microincisional IOLs are perfect platforms for toric and multifocal designs because MICS does not change the corneal astigmatism.

BAUSCH & LOMB AKREOS MI60 INTRAOCULAR LENS

Although presented by the manufacturer as an evolution from previous models, the Akreos MI60 IOL (Bausch & Lomb) is a completely new IOL (Figure 17-3). The material

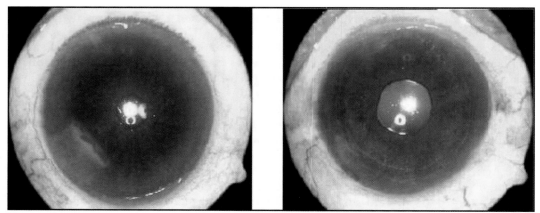

Figure 17-2. Comparison between phako foldable and bimanual MICS (B-MICS; phakonit) ThinOptX intraocular lens (IOL). The figure on the left shows a case of phako with a foldable IOL and the figure on the right shows B-MICS with a ThinOptX rollable IOL. (Photo courtesy of Dr. Agarwal's Group of Eye Hospitals and Eye Research Centre, Chennai, India.)

Figure 17-3. Microincisional Akreos MI60 intraocular lens implantation. (Photo courtesy of Dr. Agarwal's Group of Eye Hospitals and Eye Research Centre, Chennai, India.)

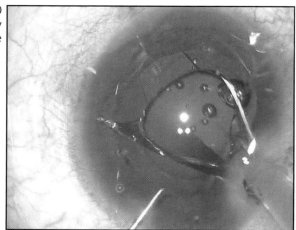

is hydrophilic acrylic with 26% water content, the total length is 10.5 to 11 mm, and the optic diameter is 5.6 to 6.2 mm, depending on the dioptric power. The optic design is neutral aspheric equiconvex. This lens has several innovative features that indicate improved understanding of ultra-small-incision IOL design. The IOL has 4 haptics that are angulated posteriorly to increase resistance to vitreous pressure and improve anteroposterior lens stability. Additionally, this thin haptic design provides 4 footplates that can curl up to prevent decentration from capsular fibrosis, thus promoting early and stable centration. When implanted in normal eyes, the Akreos MI60 IOL provides results similar to larger acrylic IOLs, with equivalent centration compared with the standard Akreos Adapt. The results in terms of refraction and optical aberrations have also been good. With this neutral aspheric microincisional IOL, postoperative higher-order aberrations are the same as the preoperative corneal surface aberrations in uncomplicated eyes. The industry calls this condition *aberration-free cataract surgery*, which means that the IOL is tolerant to decentration and may have better depth of focus than IOLs that correct larger amounts of corneal asphericity.

MICROINCISIONAL INTRAOCULAR LENSES

Table 17-1
CHARACTERISTICS OF MICROINCISIONAL IOLS THAT CAN BE IMPLANTED THROUGH SUB-2-MM INCISION*

	Acri.Tec Acri.Smart 36A	Acri.Tec Acri.Smart 46S	Acri.Tec Acri.Smart 46LC	Acri.Tec Acri.Smart 48S	Acri.Tec Acri.Smart 646TLC	Acri.Tec Acri.Smart 366D	Acri.Tec Acri.Smart 466TD	Bausch & Lomb Akreos MI60	Lenstec ZR 1000
Optic sphericity	Aspheric	Spheric	Neutral aspheric	Spheric	Bitoric aspheric	Bifocal, neutral aspheric	Bifocal, toric, neutral aspheric	Neutral aspheric	Spheric
Design	Single piece, plate haptic, anterior aspheric surface	Single piece, plate haptic, biconvex spheric surface	Single piece, plate haptic, neutral aspheric	Single piece, plate haptic, biconvex spheric surface	Single piece, plate haptic, biconvex spheric toric surface	Single piece, plate haptic, neutral aspheric anterior surface, bifocal posterior surface	Single piece, plate haptic, neutral aspheric, anterior toric surface, bifocal posterior surface	Single with four plate haptics	Single piece, plate haptic, equiconvex
Optic diameter	6 mm	6 mm	6 mm	5.5 mm	6 mm	6 mm	6 mm	6.2 mm (0 D-15 D IOL power) 6.0 mm (15.5 D-22 D IOL power) 5.6 mm (22.5 D-30 D IOL power)	5.5 mm
Overall size	11 mm	11 mm	11 mm	11 mm	11 mm	11 mm	11 mm	11 (0 D-15 D IOL power) 10.7 (15.5 D-22 D IOL power) 10.5 (22.5 D-30 D IOL power)	11 mm
Material	Hydrophilic acrylic (25% water content) with hydrophobic surface	Hydrophilic acrylic (25% water content) with hydrophobic surface	Hydrophilic acrylic (25% water content) with hydrophobic surface	Hydrophilic acrylic (25% water content) with hydrophobic surface	Hydrophilic acrylic (25% water content) with hydrophobic surface	Hydrophilic acrylic (25% water content) with hydrophobic surface	Hydrophilic acrylic (25% water content) with hydrophobic surface	Hydrophilic acrylic (26% water content)	Hydrophilic acrylic (26% water content)

*IOL indicates intraocular lens.

Lenstec ZR-1000

The ZR-1000 IOL is manufactured by Lenstec (St. Petersburg, FL), which was founded in 1992. Lenstec ZR-1000 is a UV-blocking, single-piece acrylic IOL with 2 positioning holes. It is available in a wide range from +5 to 36 diopters and in half diopter increments between +10 and +30 diopters. HumanOptics and many other European companies are developing products in this field.

Performance of Various Microincisional Intraocular Lenses

MICS can be performed using a bimanual or microcoaxial approach. Bimanual phacoemulsification has been compared with standard or microcoaxial phacoemulsification in several prospective randomized clinical trials. Both techniques are undergoing rapid development. Most studies have concentrated on the surgical aspects of bimanual surgery compared with coaxial phacoemulsification; few comparative studies have evaluated MICS IOLs specifically. The intraoperative problems associated with MICS IOLs include stretching and distortion of the corneal wound from insertion and IOL damage during insertion.[2,3] In the subsequent postoperative period, IOL decentration or folding may occur as the capsular bag fibroses, and there have been reports of very thin MICS IOLs (eg, ThinOptX IOL) tilting and decentring as the capsule fibroses after surgery.[1,4] In our study,[5] the haptic of the HumanOptics MC611MI microincisional IOL was seen to fold toward or under the optic, although this did not appear to have an effect on vision or subsequent PCO. Current micro-IOL designs that are now available appear to be stable, center well in the bag, and do not distort with capsular fibrosis.

Alió et al,[6] in a prospective nonrandomized consecutive series comprised of 30 eyes implanted with a conventional acrylic foldable (AcrySof MA60BM, Alcon), the UltraChoice 1.0 ThinOptX or the Acri.Smart 48S IO, found excellent in vivo MTF measurements with the microincisional IOLs that were comparable to conventional IOLs. The Acri.LISA 366D multifocal IOL provides a satisfactory range of uncorrected and corrected distance, intermediate and near acuity, and improved contrast sensitivity under photopic and mesopic conditions.[7] In another study, Alió et al[8] showed that the Acri.LISA 366D multifocal IOL gave good efficacy, predictability, and safety and excellent visual acuity at distance and near along with good aberration correction, Strehl ratio, and MTF values. After laser-assisted in situ keratotomy, the aspheric Acri.LISA 366D multifocal IOL provided better visual and optical quality than a spherical AcrySof SA60D3 multifocal IOL under mesopic conditions (large pupil).[9] Both multifocal IOLs provided good and comparable visual acuity at distance and near. However, the aspherical Acri.LISA multifocal IOL gives better intermediate visual acuity than the spherical AcrySof ReStor IOL in eyes that have had previous refractive surgery. This would not be surprising because the aspheric IOL will correct the increased positive corneal spherical aberration seen after myopic excimer laser treatment.[10]

Initial hopes that the thinness and flexibility of MICS IOLs would allow forward movement and focus shift of the optic in the bag to produce an accommodative element do not appear to be substantiated by clinical experience.

Posterior capsule opacification (PCO) remains the most common complication of all cataract surgery and the contribution of IOL design to the prevention of PCO is well established. The most critical IOL factor in preventing PCO is a square profile to the posterior optic edge. Most MICS IOLs are based on plate haptic designs that have not been as efficient at preventing PCO as traditional circular optic designs because lens epithelial cells tend to migrate under the plate haptic, where there is no square edge barrier (through-haptic PCO).

Our intraindividual study specifically compared the HumanOptics MC611MI microincisional IOL (not on the market any more) and the Alcon AcrySof MA60AC, which have very different designs.[5] Although both IOLs have good PCO performance overall, our results showed that the PCO performance of the MC611MI IOL was not as good as that of the AcrySof MA60AC IOL at 2 years after surgery. The difference in PCO performance between these IOLs is likely to reflect their differences in biomaterial and design with a through-haptic pattern of PCO being observed in 55% of eyes with the microincisional IOL.[5] In an ongoing, prospective, randomized study comparing the Acri.Smart 36A and Akreos MI60 microincisional IOLs, PCO was observed with these microincisional IOLs during early follow-up (unpublished data). The edge of the MI60 has since been further modified. The plate haptics or broad haptics design are the likely cause of greater PCO in the group with microincisional IOLs.

Interestingly, almost all of the microincisional IOLs currently on the market are hydrophilic acrylics, which may add to the concern of increasing PCO with these IOLs. Two prospective studies reported poor PCO performance with another MICS IOL, the ThinOptX Ultrachoice 1.0.[1,4] In a noncomparative study,[1] 64% of 50 eyes required an Nd:YAG capsulotomy for visually significant PCO after 15 months of follow-up. A comparative study[4] found that the ThinOptX IOL had worse PCO performance and, consequently, visual performance than the AcrySof MA30AC 1 year postoperatively. Poor PCO performance may thus outweigh the benefits of a smaller incision with these MICS IOLs until improvements in IOL design are made.

Summary

MICS is potentially a leap forward in the field of cataract surgery. Many companies make microincisional IOLs that can be implanted through sub-2-mm incisions, and these are likely to be increasingly popular. The combination of aspheric and multifocal technology with the microincisional IOL platform further enhances the popularity of this new technology. Comparative studies comparing the performances of these microincisional IOLs to standard IOLs are needed. Although significant achievement has already been made in this field, further refinement may be necessary to improve their PCO performance if these IOLs are to give equivalent or superior results to the existing conventional IOLs.

References

1. Prakash P, Kasaby HE, Aggarwal RK, Humfrey S. Microincision bimanual phacoemulsification and ThinOptX implantation through a 1.70 mm incision. *Eye.* 2007;21(2):177-182.
2. Cavallini GM, Campi L, Masini C, Pelloni S, Pupino A. Bimanual microphacoemulsification versus coaxial miniphacoemulsification: prospective study. *J Cataract Refract Surg.* 2007;33(3):387-392.
3. Berdahl JP, DeStafeno JJ, Kim T. Corneal wound architecture and integrity after phacoemulsification; evaluation of coaxial, microincision coaxial, and microincision bimanual techniques. *J Cataract Refract Surg.* 2007;33(3):510-515.
4. Kaya V, Özturker ZK, Özturker C, et al. ThinOptX vs AcrySof: comparison of visual and refractive results, contrast sensitivity, and the incidence of posterior capsule opacification. *Eur J Ophthalmol.* 2007;17(3):307-314.
5. Cleary G, Spalton DJ, Hancox J, Boyce J, Marshall J. Randomized intraindividual comparison of posterior capsule opacification between a microincision intraocular lens and a conventional intraocular lens. *J Cataract Refract Surg.* 2009;35(2):265-272.
6. Alió JL, Schimchak P, Montés-Micó R, Galal A. Retinal image quality after microincision intraocular lens implantation. *J Cataract Refract Surg.* 2005;31(8):1557-1560.
7. Alfonso JF, Fernández-Vega L, Señaris A, Montés-Micó R. Prospective study of the Acri.LISA bifocal intraocular lens. *J Cataract Refract Surg.* 2007;33(11):1930-1935.

8. Alió JL, Elkady B, Ortiz D, Bernabeu G. Clinical outcomes and intraocular optical quality of a diffractive multifocal intraocular lens with asymmetrical light distribution. *J Cataract Refract Surg.* 2008;34(6):942-948.
9. Fernández-Vega L, Madrid-Costa D, Alfonso JF, Montés-Micó R, Poo-López A. Optical and visual performance of diffractive intraocular lens implantation after myopic laser in situ keratomileusis. *J Cataract Refract Surg.* 2009;35(5):825-832.
10. Alfonso JF, Madrid-Costa D, Poo-López A, Montés-Micó R. Visual quality after diffractive intraocular lens implantation in eyes with previous myopic laser in situ keratomileusis. *J Cataract Refract Surg.* 2008;34(11):1848-1854.

CHAPTER 18

MICROINCISIONAL CATARACT SURGERY IN THE ERA OF REFRACTIVE CATARACT SURGERY

Robert Weinstock, MD and Neel R. Desai, MD

In recent years, cataract surgeons have witnessed dramatic growth in the level of sophistication in surgical techniques and technologies used to safely and consistently deliver optimum outcomes to a patient population with ever-increasing visual demands and expectations. This sea change has been most driven by changes in 2 key facets of the refractive-cataract surgery arena—developments in microincisional cataract surgery (MICS) techniques combined with the use of a host refractive intraocular lenses (IOL).

LENS OPTIONS FOR REFRACTIVE CATARACT SURGERY

One of the first entries to the refractive cataract surgery arena was the introduction of so-called aspheric IOL implants that have zero or negative spherical aberration. Spherical aberration occurs when light rays are overrefracted at the periphery of a lens, resulting in an area of defocused light that can degrade image quality and contrast sensitivity (Figure 18-1).[1] The optics of an aspheric lens compensate for the positive spherical aberration in a naturally prolate cornea by inducing counteracting negative spherical aberration in a manner that mimics the oblate crystalline lens in a youthful eye. Furthermore, the corneal horizontal coma is compensated for by counteracting optics within a youthful crystalline lens and are increased with a decentered IOL.[2] With aging and the development of a cataract, the counterbalancing effect of the crystalline lens on these optical aberrations is significantly reduced.[3] IOLs such as the TECNIS lens (Abbott Medical Optics, Santa Ana, CA; Figure 18-2), and the STAAR Collamer (STAAR, Monrovia, CA; Figure 18-3) achieve superior optical quality with less glare and halo and better contrast sensitivity by addressing these higher order aberrations during cataract surgery.[4]

An expanding variety of lens designs now exists to minimize or eliminate presbyopia following cataract extraction. First, several lenses incorporate multifocal designs. The Alcon ReStor SN6AD3 was the first single-piece biconvex acrylic multifocal lens with a unique apodized diffractive anterior surface. With a 13-mm overall diameter and a 6-mm optic, the lens' anterior surface possesses a 3.6-mm-diameter area containing 12 stepped zones of apodization that give it a 4 diopter add power in the lens plane and an effective 3.2 diopter add in the spectacle plane. Alcon has recently introduced the AcrySof ReStor 3.0 D IOL,

Figure 18-1. With traditional IOLs, light is more refracted at the periphery of the lens than at the center, producing positive spherical aberration. This lenticular aberration augments the existing positive aberration of a prolate cornea, resulting in reduced functional vision. (Reprinted with permission from Abbott Medical Optics, Santa Ana, CA.)

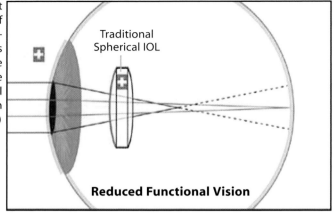

Figure 18-2. The TECNIS Acrylic IOL (left) and Silicone IOL (right) were the first lenses to incorporate wavefront-guided design to reduce spherical aberration. (Reprinted with permission from Abbott Medical Optics, Santa Ana, CA.)

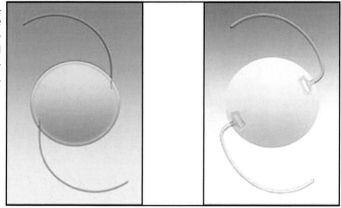

Figure 18-3. The Collamer lens utilizes an aspheric design to minimize postsurgical total spherical aberration. (Reprinted with permission from STAAR, Monrovia, CA.)

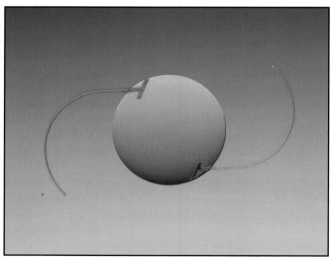

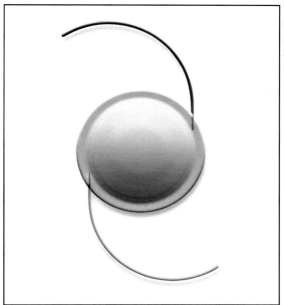

Figure 18-4. The ReZoom multifocal lens is a presbyopia correcting lens with 5 refractive optical zones. (Reprinted with permission from Abbott Medical Optics, Santa Ana, CA.)

which has an effective add of 2.5 diopters in the spectacle plane. To preserve optical quality, the number of steps within the apodized zone was reduced to 9 diffractive steps. These new generations of the Alcon ReStor also incorporate asphericity to greatly reduce complaints of glare, halo, and decreased contrast sensitivity. The optic and haptics have a square-edge design to minimize posterior capsular opacification.[5]

The ReZoom IOL (Figure 18-4) by Abbott Medical Optics is a 13.0-mm-diameter 3-piece hydrophobic acrylic multifocal IOL that distributes light over 5 refractive optical zones, with a central-distance dominant zone within a 6.0-mm optic to provide a near add of 3.5 diopters at the lens plane and an effective 2.85 diopters of add in the spectacle plane. The newer TECNIS Multifocal lens (Figure 18-5) is an aspheric, fully diffractive multifocal lens providing a +4.0 diopter near add in the IOL plane and 3.2 diopters in the spectacle plane. The TECNIS multifocal design is unique in that it covers the entire optic and distributes light equally to all optical zones and ranges of vision, thus providing patients with excellent reading vision with some independence of lighting conditions and pupil size.

The Crystalens AT50 (Bausch & Lomb, Aliso Viejo, CA; Figure 18-6) accommodating IOL aims to restore a full range of vision using a 5.0-mm monofocal silicone optic built on a flexible plate platform to mimic true accommodation with contraction of the ciliary muscle. The lens design may also benefit from sitting further posteriorly in the capsular bag and thus closer to the nodal point of the eye, resulting in greater depth of focus. The Crystalens HD incorporates a unique polyspheric optic with a single central area on the anterior surface with an additional 1.0 diopter of increased power to aid near vision in the nondominant eye. This polyspheric design is distinguished from other multifocal IOLs that rely on simultaneous retinal projections that require significant neuroadaptation. The blended design of the extra single near focal point on the Crystalens HD lens increases the static depth of field to expand the effective range of accommodation in the range of object vergence between infiniti and 2.0 diopters.[6] With their unique designs, the Crystalens and Crystalens HD achieve a full range of vision for patients that is intuitively similar to the vision of their youth.

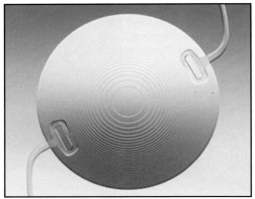

Figure 18-5. The TECNIS Multifocal lens is an aspheric, fully diffractive multifocal lens providing +3.2 diopters of near add in the spectacle plane. (Reprinted with permission from Abbott Medical Optics, Santa Ana, CA.)

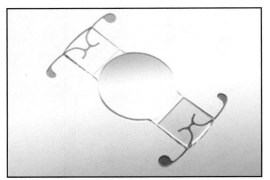

Figure 18-6. The Crystalens AT50 is an accommodating intraocular lens for the correction of presbyopia. The Crystalens HD incorporates a polyspheric design on the anterior surface that gives this accommodating lens an additional +1.0 near add power, intended for implantation in the non-dominant eye. (Reprinted with permission from Bausch & Lomb, Aliso Viejo, CA.)

In addition to the currently available presbyopia-correcting options described, several IOL design options exist for the correction of astigmatism. The STAAR Toric IOL (Figure 18-7) is a silicone plate toric lens available in 2 cylindrical powers. The 2.0 diopter cylinder lens produces 1.5 diopters of correction in the corneal plane and has an overall length of 11.2 mm. Also available is a lens with 3.5 diopters of cylindrical correction in the lens plane, producing 2.3 diopters of cylindrical correction in the corneal plane. Toric lenses offered by Alcon are based on the familiar AcrySof single-piece acrylic platform that naturally resists rotation due to its tacky nature. With cylindrical corrections in the IOL plane of 1.5 diopters in the T3 model, 2.25 diopters in the T4 model, and 3.00 diopters in the T5 model, the lens is able to achieve 1.03 diopters, 1.55 diopters, and 2.06 diopters of cylindrical correction in the corneal plane, respectively.

Multifocal toric IOLs, though still not available in the United States, are on the horizon and promise to further expand the options for patients. Rayner (Hove, East Sussex, UK) and Carl Zeiss Meditec (Jena, Germany) are forging ahead in this field. Of particular interest is the Acri.LISA toric multifocal from Carl Zeiss Meditec, which is inserted through a 1.6-mm incision, making it an exciting new option in the MICS arena.

For each of these modern lens options, however, the technology will only be as good as the techniques used to deploy them with regard to final visual outcomes. The importance of each critical step of cataract removal and lens implantation is exponentially magnified with these lenses. Common pitfalls with their use can be easily avoided with the use of equally sophisticated surgical techniques such as MICS along the way.

Using Microincisional Cataract Surgery to Achieve Optimum Outcomes With Advanced Intraocular Lenses

Wound construction in MICS constitutes more than just the making of smaller wounds for the sake of making smaller wounds. Several distinct advantages important to the use of premium IOLs arise from our ability to construct small, symmetric, and astigmatically neutral wounds. First, the flared trapezoidal blade designs create a wound with a wider

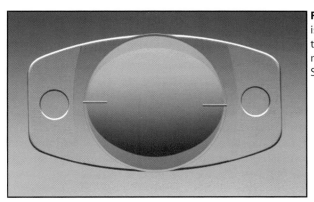

Figure 18-7. The STAAR toric intraocular lens is a silicone plate-haptic lens for the correction of up to 2.3 diopters of corneal astigmatism. (Reprinted with permission from STAAR, Monrovia, CA.)

external aperture and narrow 1.4-mm internal width. Not only does this architecture limit fluid and viscoelastics egress during the procedure, but it improves maneuverability through the wounds. Avoidance of a tight "oar-lock" with excessive pressure within the wound is critical in the prevention of wound burn.[7] Limiting fluid egress with smaller wounds naturally makes for a more stable chamber and hence limits how much irrigation fluid across the endothelium is required to maintain the chamber.

Another distinct advantage of MICS has to do with the flexibility of wound placement. Surgeons who plan to correct astigmatism on the corneal plane with limbal relaxing incisions or astigmatic keratectomies can choose to place wounds comfortably outside of the areas of intended incisional correction to avoid interference or intersection of wounds. Surgeons may also choose to place one wound that will later be enlarged for lens insertion on the steep axis. The direction of enlargement can also be customized. These advantages are particularly noticeable in patients who have had prior radial keratotomy, in which avoidance of intersecting incisions is critically important.

Finally, with biaxial microincisional surgery, the dual equally sized wounds also allow a surgeon to switch the irrigating chopper and aspirating handpieces from hand to hand, allowing full 360-degree access to nuclear fragments and cortical material. This feature of biaxial surgery is particularly beneficial when working subincisionally, where a coaxial instrument's irrigating ports may exit the eye, leading to chamber collapse and risk of posterior capsular tears. Hence, wound construction and placement in MICS can be utilized to enhance successful astigmatic correction that is critical to optimizing patients' visual outcomes with these sophisticated lenses and facilitates safe and ergonomic removal of all lens material.

The advantages of biaxial microincision phacoemulsification are most readily noticed during nucleus and cortical removal. When nuclear fragments or cortical material are located in a subincisional position, coaxial techniques require the whole handpiece to be partially withdrawn from the wound, placing the irrigation ports either within the clear corneal wound or dangerously outside of it, risking chamber collapse, anterior vaulting of the posterior capsule, and capsular tears with vitreous prolapse. With younger patients seeking refractive lens replacement and cataract patients expecting excellent visual results from advanced lens technologies, the stakes are too high to take such risks. Bimanual MICS (B-MICS) minimizes these risks by separating irrigation from aspiration. Hence, fluidic stability within the anterior chamber remains constant regardless of where the aspiration port is positioned, even when accessing subincisional cortical material. Also unlike coaxial, larger incision surgery, biaxial microincision techniques allow a surgeon to switch irrigation and aspiration instruments from hand to hand because the wounds are equally sized. This further expands the safe range of maneuverability within the eye. Furthermore, nuclear fragments and cortical material can be easily manipulated and the posterior capsule better protected by the ability to independently direct irrigation currents toward the posterior capsule or peripheral capsule.

Complete and careful cortical removal and capsular polishing, as afforded by biaxial MICS, is essential when implanting premium advanced IOLs. Multifocal lenses like the Alcon ReStor, Abbott Medical Optics ReZoom, and TECNIS Multifocal render patients particularly sensitive to relatively low levels of posterior capsular opacification that can be minimized with careful intraoperative techniques as described.[8] Retained cortical material in the capsular periphery, excessive Soemmering's ring formation, or capsular retention syndrome can significantly dislocate any lens but with greater detrimental impact to multifocal lenses, toric lenses, and accommodating lenses due to their advanced and unique optics.

Biaxial also renders cases of intraoperative floppy iris syndrome (IFIS) and small-pupil cases more routine rather than fraught with the difficulty and potential complications seen with conventional coaxial techniques.[9] IFIS is commonly associated with medications like tamsolusin and nonselective α1-adrenergic antagonists like terazosin.[10] However, other pharmaceutical classes may be loosely implicated, including angiotensin antagonists such as losartan and lisinopril, muscle relaxants such as orphenadrine and metaxalone, and herbal supplements like saw palmetto.[11] In coaxial surgery, with each anterior-to-posterior, side-to-side, or rotational movement of the handpiece, the directional fluidics change and result in turbulence, iris billowing, pupillary constriction, and poor visualization. In such cases, biaxial microincision surgery is a far superior technique versus other modalities due to the ability to keep the directional flow of irrigation above or at the iris plane to minimize turbulence and billowing of the iris. With any small-pupil case, the 20-gauge or smaller instruments inherently have a smaller profile and provide better control and visualization.

Microincisional Cataract Surgery Intraocular Lenses

Surgeons reluctant to convert to biaxial microincision surgery, despite the clear advantages, often cite the need to enlarge a small 1.2-mm incision to accommodate insertion of most commonly available IOLs through a 2.2- to 2.8-mm incision. However, as the advantages of biaxial microincision techniques become apparent, especially in the era of advanced implants and concomitant high-stakes expectations, other lens options for small-incision insertion will become available within the United States and other markets. Carl Zeiss has the Acri.Tec lens (Figure 18-8). Newer lenses such as the TECNIS one-piece IOL, when used with the Duckworth & Kent (Hertfordshire, UK) inserter, and the Akreos hydrophilic acrylic IOL (Bausch & Lomb; approved by the US Food and Drug Administration in 2008) can be inserted through 2.0-mm incisions (Figures 18-9 and 18-10).

Light Adjustable Lens

One of the most exciting technologies is the light adjustable lens (LAL; Calhoun Vision, Pasadena, CA). The LAL is designed to allow for postoperative refinements of lens power in situ. The current design of the LAL is a foldable 3-piece IOL with a cross-linked silicone polymer matrix and a homogeneously embedded photosensitive macromer. The application of near-ultraviolet light to a portion of the lens optic results in polymerization of the photosensitive macromers and precise changes in lens power through a mechanism of macromer migration into polymerized regions and subsequent changes in lens thickness (Figure 18-11).

MICROINCISIONAL CATARACT SURGERY IN THE ERA OF REFRACTIVE CATARACT SURGERY

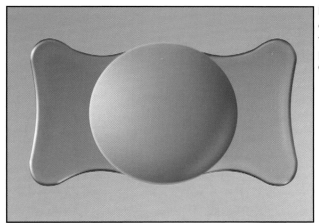

Figure 18-8. The Acri.Tec lens from is an example of a lens that can be inserted through microincisions. (Reprinted with permission from Carl Zeiss Meditec, Jena, Germany.)

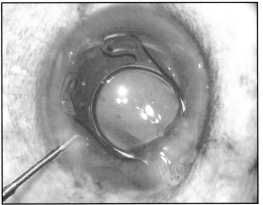

Figure 18-9. The Akreos intraocular lens from Bausch & Lomb. (Photo courtesy of Dr. Agarwal's Group of Eye Hospitals and Eye Research Centre, Chennai, India.)

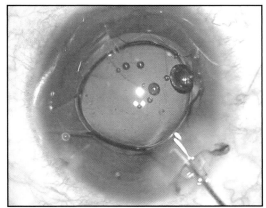

Figure 18-10. Akreos MI 60 intraocular lens from Bausch & Lomb for MICS. (Photo courtesy of Dr. Agarwal's Group of Eye Hospitals and Eye Research Centre, Chennai, India.)

WAVETEC ORANGE

Other technologies will also be used synergistically with advanced implants and MICS to provide even greater levels of sophistication and care. Our practice in Largo, FL, is one of the first in the world to employ the ORange (WaveTec Vision, Aliso Viejo, CA), a pioneering intraoperative aberrometer that provides intraoperative wavefront-based analysis of refraction. We already find this especially useful in the planning and execution of astigmatic corrections on the corneal plane as well as the precise positioning of toric implants. This technology shows great promise in providing intraoperative feedback to surgeons challenged with an ever-increasing population of postrefractive surgery cataract patients.

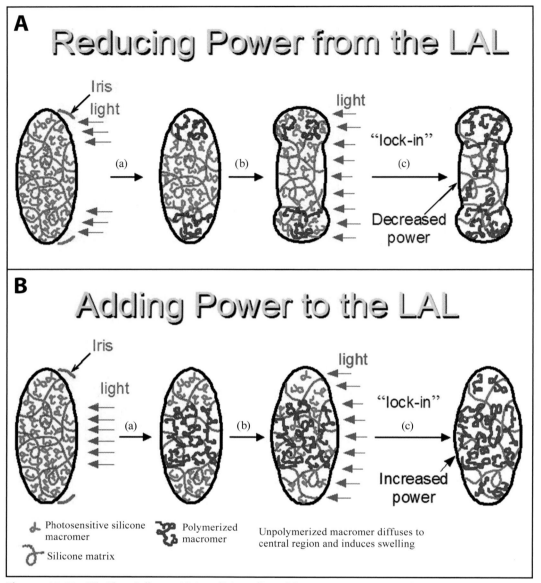

Figure 18-11. (A) The Calhoun Vision light adjustable IOL. Cross-sectional schematic illustration of mechanism for treating myopic correction. (a) Selective irradiation of peripheral portion of lens polymerizes macromer, creating a chemical gradient between irradiated and nonirradiated regions; (b) macromer from the central zone diffuses peripherally leading to swelling of the peripheral lens; (c) irradiation of the entire lens polymerizes the remaining macromer and "locks-in" the new lens shape with less power.[9] (B) Cross-sectional schematic illustration of mechanism for treating hyperopic correction. (a) Selective irradiation of central portion of lens polymerizes macromer, creating a chemical gradient between irradiated and nonirradiated regions; (b) in order to reestablish equilibrium, macromer from the peripheral lens diffuses into the central irradiated region, leading to swelling of the central zone; (c) irradiation of the entire lens polymerizes the remaining macromer and "locks-in" the new lens shape.[9] (Reprinted with permission from Agarwal A. *Phaco Nightmares: Conquering Cataract Catastrophes.* Thorofare, NJ: SLACK Incorporated; 2006.)

Summary

Surgeons who make the transition to B-MICS will find that the level of sophistication, intraoperative control, fluid dynamics, and overall safety of the procedure far exceeds that seen with coaxial large incision surgery. MICS techniques will help the surgeon capitalize on every critical step of the procedure to reach consistently excellent outcomes. The capabilities of these techniques blend perfectly with the requirements of success with advanced implants and the goal and desire to meet and exceed patient expectations.

References

1. Atchison D, Smith G. *Optics of the Human Eye*. Edinburgh, UK: Butterworth-Heinemann; 2000.
2. Bellucci R, Morselli S, Pucci V. Spherical aberration and coma with an aspherical and a spherical intraocular lens in normal age-matched eyes. *J Cataract Refract Surg*. 2007;33(2):203-209.
3. Alío JL, Schimchak P, Negri HP, Montés-Micó R. Crystalline lens optical dysfunction through aging. *Ophthalmology*. 2005;112(11):2022-2029.
4. Ruttig NJ, Jancevski M, Shah SA. Evaluating wavefront analysis application in intraocular lens placement. *Curr Opin Ophthalmol*. 2008;19(4):309-313.
5. Buehl W, Findl O. Effect of intraocular lens design on posterior capsule opacification [Review]. *J Cataract Refract Surg*. 2008;34(11):1976-1985.
6. Cummings JS. Polyspheric accomodating intraocular lens. United States Patent Application Publication; January 2008.
7. Sippel KC, Pineda R, Jr. Phacoemulsification and thermal wound injury. *Semin Ophthalmol*. 2002;17(3-4):102-109.
8. Cionni R. Strategies for multifocal IOLs. Paper presented at: ASCRS Symposium on Cataract, IOL and Refractive Surgery; April 4-9, 2008; Chicago, IL.
9. Agarwal A. *Bimanual Phaco: Mastering the Phakonit/MICS Technique*. Thorofare, NJ: SLACK Incorporated; 2004.
10. Chang DF, Campbell JR. Intraoperative floppy iris syndrome associated with tamsulosin. *J Cataract Refract Surg*. 2005;31(4):664-673.
11. Neff KD, Sandoval HP, Fernández de Castro LE, Nowacki AS, Vroman DT, Solomon KD. Factors associated with intraoperative floppy iris syndrome. *Ophthalmology*. 2009;116(4):658-663.

CHAPTER 19

POSTERIOR CAPSULAR RUPTURE AND ITS MANAGEMENT

Soosan Jacob, MS, FRCS, FERC, Dip NB; Dhivya Ashok Kumar, MD; Kaladevi Satish, MS; Clement K. Chan, MD, FACS; and Amar Agarwal, MS, FRCS, FRCOphth

Any breach in the continuity of the posterior capsule is defined as a *posterior capsule tear*. Intrasurgical posterior capsule tears are the most common and can occur during any stage of cataract surgery.[1-3] The incidence of posterior capsule complications is related to the type of cataract and conditions of the eye, increases with the grade of difficulty of the case, and furthermore is influenced by the level of experience of the surgeon. Timely recognition and a planned management, depending upon the stage of surgery during which the posterior capsule tear has occurred, is required to ensure an optimal visual outcome.

STEPS FOR MANAGEMENT OF POSTERIOR CAPSULE RUPTURE

The surgeon should be aware of the signs (Table 19-1) of posterior capsular tear. Posterior capsule tears can occur during any stage of phacoemulsification surgery (Figure 19-1). They occur most frequently during the stage of nuclear emulsification, as reported by Mulhern et al[4] (49%) and Osher et al,[5] and during irrigation/aspiration, as reported by Gimbel et al.[6]

Three possible situations can happen in a posterior capsule rent[7]:

1. Posterior capsule tear with hyaloid face intact and nuclear material present
2. Posterior capsule tear with hyaloid face ruptured without luxation of nuclear material into vitreous
3. Posterior capsule tear with hyaloid face ruptured and luxation of nuclear material into vitreous

Immediate precautions are to be taken not to further hydrate the vitreous and not to increase the size of the posterior capsule rupture (PCR). Conventional management consists of the prevention of a mixture of cortical matter with vitreous, dry aspiration, and anterior vitrectomy, if required. In addition, during phacoemulsification, low flow rate, high vacuum, and low ultrasound are advocated if a posterior capsule tear occurs.

Table 19-1
SIGNS OF POSTERIOR CAPSULAR RUPTURE
1. Sudden deepening of the chamber, with momentary expansion of the pupil
2. Sudden, transitory appearance of a clear red reflex peripherally
3. Apparent inability to rotate a previously mobile nucleus
4. Excessive lateral mobility or displacement of the nucleus
5. Excessive tipping of one pole of the nucleus
6. Partial descent of the nucleus into the anterior vitreous space
7. "Pupil snap sign"—sudden marked pupil constriction after hydro dissection

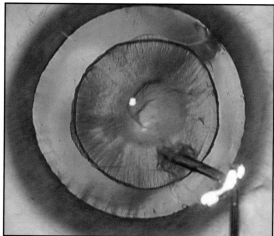

Figure 19-1. Hydrodelineation being performed in a posterior polar cataract.

REDUCE THE PARAMETERS

Lowering aspiration flow rate and decreasing the vacuum will control surge and will allow the bottle to be lowered, diminishing turbulence inside the eye. If the nucleus is soft, only a small residual amount remains, and there is no vitreous prolapse, the procedure may be continued. If vitreous is already present, special care must be taken for preventing additional vitreous prolapse into the anterior chamber or to the wound. Small residual nucleus or cortex can be emulsified by bringing it out of the capsular bag for emulsification in the anterior chamber with viscoelastic underneath the corneal endothelium. In case of a small PCR and minimal residual nucleus (Figure 19-2), a dispersive viscoelastic is injected to plug the posterior capsule tear. Subsequently, the nuclear material is moved into the anterior chamber with a spatula and emulsified. The recommended parameters are low bottle height (20-40 cm above the patient's head), low flow rate (10-15 cc/min), high vacuum (120-200 mm Hg), and low ultrasound (20%-40%).

DRY CORTICAL ASPIRATION

If there is only a small amount or no vitreous prolapse in the presence of a small capsular rent, a dry cortical aspiration with a 23-gauge cannula can be performed.

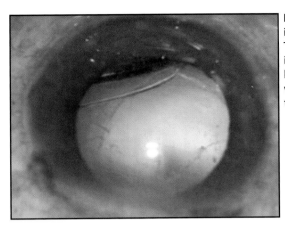

Figure 19-2. Posterior capsular rupture. Note the intraocular lens sinking into the vitreous cavity. The white reflex indicates nuclear fragments also in the vitreous cavity. This patient was managed by vitrectomy, FAVIT (FA = fallen, VIT = vitreous; which is removal of the nuclear fragments), and the intraocular lens repositioned in the sulcus.

VISCOEXPRESSION

Viscoexpression is a method of removal of the residual nucleus by injecting viscoelastic underneath the nucleus to support it and the nucleus is expressed along with the viscoelastic.

CONVERSION TO EXTRACAPSULAR CATARACT EXTRACTION

If there is a sizeable amount of residual nucleus, it is advisable to convert to a large incision extracapsular cataract extraction to minimize the possibility of a dropped nucleus.

ANTERIOR BIMANUAL VITRECTOMY

Bimanual vitrectomy (Figure 19-3) is done in eyes with vitreous prolapse. Use a 23-gauge irrigating cannula via the side port after extending the side-port incision. The irrigation bottle is positioned at the appropriate height to maintain the anterior chamber during vitrectomy. Vitrectomy should be performed with a cutting rate of 500 to 800 cuts per minute, an aspiration flow rate of 20 cc/min, and a vacuum of 150 to 200 mm Hg.

ANTERIOR CHAMBER CLEARED OF VITREOUS

Vitrectomy is continued in the anterior chamber and the pupillary plane. A rod can be introduced into the anterior chamber to check the presence of any vitreous traction and the same should be released. Complete removal of the vitreous from the anterior chamber can be confirmed if you see a circular, mobile pupil (Figure 19-4) and complete air bubble in the anterior chamber. The usage of the fiber of an endoilluminator and dimming the room lights and microscope lights may be useful in cases of doubt in order to identify vitreous strands. Another useful measure is the use of purified triamcinolone acetate suspension (triamcinolone acetonide; Kenalog) to identify the vitreous described by Peyman.[8] Kenalog particles remain trapped on and within the vitreous gel, making it clearly visible.[9]

SUTURE THE WOUND

In cases with vitreous loss with PCR, it is recommended to suture the corneal wound as a prophylaxis to prevent infection. Remove any residual vitreous in the incision site in the main and side port with a vitrector or manually with Vannas scissors. If necessary, insert a rod via the side port and pass it over the surface of the iris to release them.

Figure 19-3. Bimanual vitrectomy is being performed in a posterior capsular tear with vitreous prolapse.

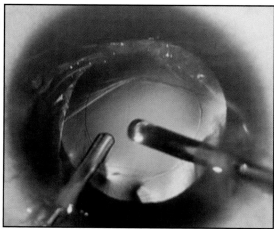

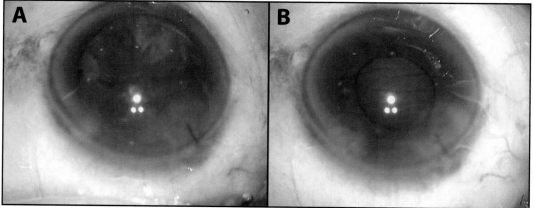

Figure 19-4. Clinical photograph showing the change in the anterior chamber after complete removal of the vitreous from the anterior chamber. (A) Before vitrectomy. (B) After vitrectomy.

INTRAOCULAR LENS IMPLANTATION

Depending upon the state of the capsular bag and rhexis, an intraocular lens (IOL) is implanted (Table 19-2).

IN THE BAG

In the presence of a posterior capsule tear with good capsular bag, the IOL can be placed in the bag. For a small PCR with no vitreous loss and good capsular bag, a foldable IOL can be placed.

IN THE SULCUS

If the rent is large and the capsular rim is available, the IOL can be placed in the sulcus. The rigid IOL can be placed in the sulcus in a large PCR over the residual anterior capsular rim with McPherson forceps (Katena, Denville, NJ) holding the optic. The "chopstick technique" is another method of placing an IOL in the sulcus, which uses the new chopstick forceps (Agarwal-Katena forceps, Katena; Figure 19-5) for IOL implantation. This chopstick technique refers to the IOL being held between 2 flanges of the forceps. The advantage

POSTERIOR CAPSULAR RUPTURE AND ITS MANAGEMENT

Table 19-2

IOL IMPLANTATION IN PCR

1. Insertion and rotation of the IOL should always be away from the area of capsule tear.
2. The long axis of the IOL should cross the meridian of the posterior capsule tear.
3. Eyes with (< 6mm) PCR with no vitreous loss, IOL can be placed in the capsular bag.
4. In the presence of a posterior capsule tear (> 6mm) with adequate anterior capsule rim, an IOL can be placed in the sulcus.
5. In deficient capsules, glued IOL is a promising technique without complications of sutured scleral fixated or anterior chamber IOL.

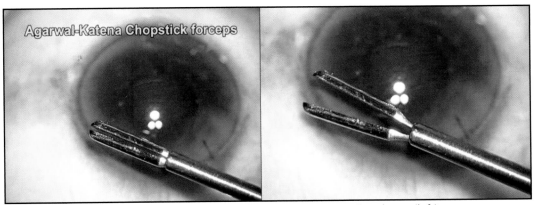

Figure 19-5. Photograph of an Agarwal-Katena forceps. Reverse opening shown (left).

is the smooth placement of the IOL in the sulcus without excess manipulation. Moreover, the IOL implantation is more controlled (Figure 19-6) with this forceps compared to other methods. For a small PCR with no vitreous loss and good capsular bag, a foldable IOL can be placed (Figure 19-7). The chopstick forceps is especially helpful when implanting a PC IOL in the sulcus in cases that have a large anterior capsular rhexis, a small pupil in which the rhexis margin is not seen, or in which the anterior rhexis margin is torn. In such cases, one can wrongly implant the PC IOL posterior to the anterior capsular rhexis rather than anterior to it. One should also remember not to implant a single-piece acrylic lens in such cases because it is better to implant a 3-piece IOL.

In eyes with intraoperative miosis with PCR, an IOL can be implanted with the pupil expansion using Agarwal's modified Malyugin ring (MicroSurgical Technology, Redmond, WA) method (Figure 19-8). In this method,[10] a 6-0 polyglactic suture is placed in the leading scroll of the Malyugin ring and injected into the pupillary plane (Figure 19-9). The end of the suture stays at the main port incision. Once in place, the ring produces a stable mydriasis of about 6.0 mm. An IOL can then be implanted easily in the sulcus with visualization. This prevents the inadvertent dropping of the iris expander into the vitreous during intraoperative manipulation.

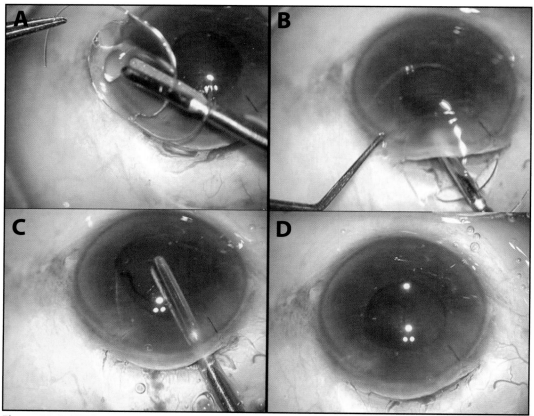

Figure 19-6. (A) The 6.5-mm PMMA rigid IOL being held between 2 flanges of the forceps. (B) IOL is being introduced through the limbal incision. (C) IOL is positioned in the sulcus. (D) IOL is well centered.

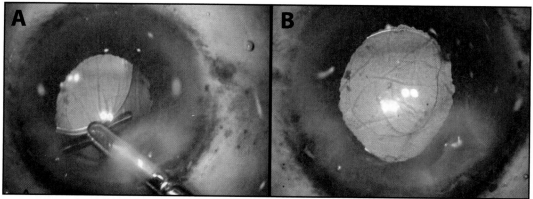

Figure 19-7. (A) Foldable IOL is placed with Agarwal-Katena forceps into the sulcus. (B) IOL well centered on the capsular rim.

POSTERIOR CAPSULAR RUPTURE AND ITS MANAGEMENT

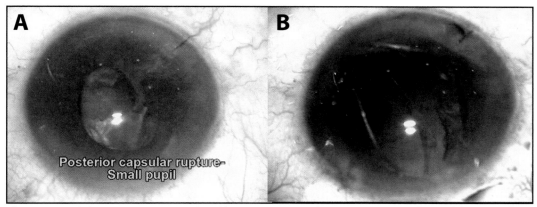

Figure 19-8. (A) Intraoperative miosis with posterior capsular tear. (B) Agarwal's modification of the Malyugin ring iris expansion: a 6-0 polyglactic vicryl suture is passed in the leading scroll of the ring and injected. The end of the suture stays at the main port incision.

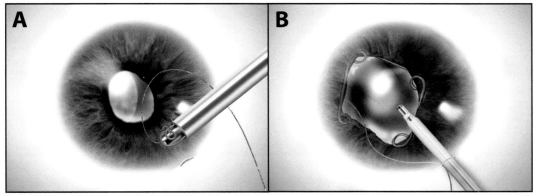

Figure 19-9. Illustration depicting the Agarwal modification of the Malyugin ring for cases with small pupil with a posterior capsular rupture. (A) 6-0 Suture tied to the ring. (B) Malyugin ring in place in the pupil. The suture can be pulled if the ring begins to fall into the vitreous. (Photo courtesy of Dr. Agarwal's Group of Eye Hospitals and Eye Research Centre, Chennai, India.)

GLUED INTRAOCULAR LENS

Recently, glued IOL[11-13] is easily performed in such cases with deficient posterior capsules. Two partial-thickness limbal-based scleral flaps about 2.5 mm × 3 mm are created exactly 180 degrees diagonally apart (Figure 19-10) and about 1.5 mm from the limbus. This is followed by vitrectomy via pars plana or anterior route to remove all vitreous traction. Two straight sclerotomies with a 22-gauge needle are made about 1.5 mm from the limbus under the existing scleral flaps. A scleral tunnel incision is then prepared for introducing the IOL. While the IOL is being placed using a McPherson forceps, an end-gripping 25-gauge microrhexis forceps (MicroSurgical Technology) is passed through the inferior sclerotomy. The tip of the leading haptic is then grasped with the microrhexis forceps, pulled through the inferior sclerotomy following the curve of the haptic, and externalized under the inferior scleral flap. Similarly, the trailing haptic is externalized through the superior sclerotomy under the scleral flap. The limbal wound is sutured with 10-0 monofilament nylon. The tip of the haptics are then tucked inside a scleral tunnel made with a 26-gauge needle at the point of extension. Scleral flaps are closed with fibrin glue.

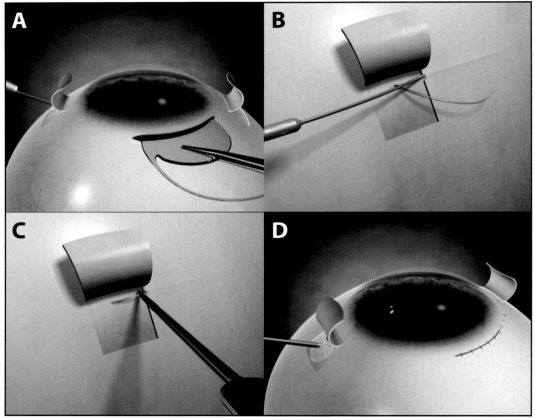

Figure 19-10. (A) Two partial-thickness scleral flaps made 180 degrees apart and a 3-piece foldable/nonfoldable IOL is introduced through the limbal incision while the haptic is externalized through the sclerotomy beneath the flaps. (B) Scleral tunnel created with 26-gauge needle. (C) Intraocular lens haptic is tucked into the tunnel. (D) Fibrin glue is used to close the scleral flaps. (Photo courtesy of Dr. Agarwal's Group of Eye Hospitals and Eye Research Centre, Chennai, India.)

The anterior chamber maintainer or the infusion cannula is removed. The conjunctiva is also closed with the same fibrin glue. The lenses that are preferred for the glued IOL technique are 3-piece foldable IOLs. The advantage over a single-piece nonfoldable IOL is that the optic haptic junction does not crack when you flex the haptic.

Scleral fixated posterior chamber lenses and anterior chamber IOLs[14,15] can also be implanted when the posterior capsule tear is large.

DROP IN VITREOUS

A large posterior capsular tear or zonular dialysis[3] can cause intraoperative nucleus drop. Selected cases in which the displaced lens material is small (less than 5% to 10% of lens volume) or in which there is little or no intraocular inflammation and intraocular pressure is easily controlled with topical medications. Nucleus segments greater than one-fourth of the total should be removed by vitrectomy because of the risk for chronic inflammation and secondary glaucoma. Pars plana vitrectomy with or without phacofragmatome is performed. Perfluorocarbon can be used in selected cases. FAVIT technique—a technique described by Agarwal et al—can also be used.[1]

Sequelae After Posterior Capsular Rupture

* Vitreous traction: Incomplete vitrectomy can produce dynamic traction on the retina, leading to retinal breaks
* Retinal detachment: Undetected long-standing vitreous traction progresses to retinal break and detachment
* Macular edema: Manipulation of vitreous will increase not only the traction transmitted to the retina, but the inflammation in the posterior segment and the risk of macular edema
* Vitritis: Overenthusiastic use of viscoelastic into the vitreous can lead to sterile inflammation. Dropped minimal residual cortex can also present with postoperative vitritis
* IOL-related complications: An improperly placed IOL in the sulcus can lead to lens-induced astigmatism and tilt

Summary

The occurrence of a posterior capsule tear during cataract surgery is one of the most serious complications. It is important for a surgeon to diagnose the occurrence of a posterior capsule tear at an early stage to avoid further enlargement of the tear and associated vitreous complications. The primary goal of all of the maneuvers is to remove the remaining nucleus, epinucleus, and as much cortex as possible without causing vitreoretinal traction.

References

1. Agarwal A. *Phaco Nightmares; Conquering Cataract Catastrophes*. Thorofare, NJ: SLACK Incorporated; 2006.
2. Agarwal S, Agarwal A, Agarwal A. *Phacoemulsification*. 3rd ed. Delhi, India: Jaypee Brothers; 2004.
3. Fishkind WJ. Facing Down the 5 Most Common Cataract Complications. *Review of Ophthalmology*. October 2001.
4. Mulhern M, Kelly G, Barry P. Effects of posterior capsular disruption on the outcome of phacoemulsification surgery. *Br J Ophthalmol*. 1995;79(12):1133-1137.
5. Osher RH, Cionni RJ. The torn posterior capsule: its intraoperative behaviour, surgical management and long term consequences. *J Cataract Refract Surg*. 1990;16(4):490-494.
6. Gimbel HV. Posterior capsular tears during phacoemulsification—causes, prevention and management. *Eur J Refract Surg*. 1990;2:639.
7. Vajpayee RB, Sharma N, Dada T, Gupta V, Kumar A, Dada VK. Management of posterior capsule tears. *Surv Ophthal*. 2001;45:473-488.
8. Peyman GA, Cheema R, Conway MD, Fang T. Triamcinolone acetonide as an aid to visualization of the vitreous and the posterior hyaloid during pars plana vitrectomy. *Retina*. 2000;20(5):554-555.
9. Burk SE, Da Mata AP, Snyder ME, Schneider S, Osher RH, Cionni RJ. Visualizing vitreous using Kenalog suspension. *J Cataract Refract Surg*. 2003;29(4):645-651.
10. Agarwal A, Malyugin B, Kumar DA, Jacob S, Agarwal A, Laks L. Modified Malyugin ring iris expansion technique in small-pupil cataract surgery with posterior capsule defect. *J Cataract Refract Surg*. 2008;34(5):724-726.
11. Agarwal A, Kumar DA, Jacob S, Baid C, Agarwal A, Srinivasan S. Fibrin glue-assisted sutureless posterior chamber intraocular lens implantation in eyes with deficient posterior capsules. *J Cataract Refract Surg*. 2008;34(9):1433-1438.
12. Falavarjani KG, Modarres M, Foroutan A, Bakhtiari P. Fibrin glue-assisted sutureless scleral fixation [Reply to letter]. *J Cataract Refract Surg*. 2009;35(5):795-796.
13. Prakash G, Kumar DA, Jacob S, Kumar S, Agarwal A, Agarwal A. Anterior segment optical coherence tomography–aided diagnosis and primary posterior chamber intraocular lens implantation with fibrin glue in traumatic phacocele with scleral perforation. *J Cataract Refract Surg*. 2009;35(4):782-784.

14. Bleckmann H, Kaczmarek U. Functional results of posterior chamber lens implantation with scleral fixation. *J Cataract Refract Surg*. 1994;20(3):321-326.
15. Numa A, Nakamura J, Takashima M, Kani K. Long-term corneal endothelial changes after intraocular lens implantation. Anterior vs posterior chamber lenses. *Jpn J Ophthalmol*. 1993;37(1):78-87.

FINANCIAL DISCLOSURES

Dr. Athiya Agarwal has no financial or proprietary interest in the materials presented herein.

Dr. George H. H. Beiko is a consultant for Abbott Medical Optics.

Dr. Clement K. Chan is a consultant for Allergan, Genentech, Regeneron, SightPath, ThromboGenics, Alimera Sciences, and the National Institutes of Health.

Dr. Prashaant Chaudhry has no financial or proprietary interest in the materials presented herein.

Dr. Elizabeth A. Davis is a consultant for Abbott Medical Optics, ISTA, Bausch & Lomb, and Inspire. She is a speaker for Allergan. She is owner of Refractec.

Dr. Neel R. Desai has not disclosed any relevant financial relationships.

Dr. Uday Devgan has no financial or proprietary interest in the materials presented herein.

Dr. Terence M. Devine has no financial or proprietary interest in the materials presented herein.

Dr. I. Howard Fine is a consultant for Abbott Medical Optics, Bausch & Lomb, iScience, Carl Zeiss Meditec, and Omeros Corporation. He has received travel and research support from Alcon, Eyeonics, STAAR Surgical, and Rayner.

Dr. William J. Fishkind is a consultant for Abbott Medical Optics and LENSAR. He has received royalties from Theime Publishers.

Mr. Kelly J. Grimes has no financial or proprietary interest in the materials presented herein.

Dr. David R. Hardten is a consultant for Abbott Medical Optics.

Dr. Bonnie An Henderson is a consultant for Alcon labs and ISTA Pharmaceuticals.

Dr. Richard S. Hoffman has no financial or proprietary interest in the materials presented herein.

Dr. Soosan Jacob has no financial or proprietary interest in the materials presented herein.

Dr. Dhivya Ashok Kumar has no financial or proprietary interest in the materials presented herein.

Dr. Dennis C. Lu has no financial or proprietary interest in the materials presented herein.

Dr. Archana Nair has no financial or proprietary interest in the materials presented herein.

Dr. Vidya Nair has no financial or proprietary interest in the materials presented herein.

Dr. Mayank A. Nanavaty has no financial or proprietary interest in the materials presented herein.

Dr. Smita Narsimhan has no financial or proprietary interest in the materials presented herein.

FINANCIAL DISCLOSURES

Dr. Richard Packard is a consultant for Alcon, Bausch & Lomb, Abbott Medical Optics, MicroSurgical Technology, and Core Surgical.

Dr. Mark Packer is a consultant for Abbott Medical Optics, Advanced Vision Science, Bausch & Lomb, Celgene Cellular Therapeutics, Carl Zeiss Surgical, General Electric Company, Haag-Streit USA, Rayner Intraocular Lenses, Transcend Medical, TrueVision Systems, Visiogen, and WaveTec Vision Systems. He also holds stock options with TrueVision Systems, Visiogen, and WaveTec Vision Systems.

Dr. Arturo Pèrez-Arteaga has no financial or proprietary interest in the materials presented herein.

Dr. Gaurav Prakash has no financial or proprietary interest in the materials presented herein.

Dr. Shetal M. Raj has no financial or proprietary interest in the materials presented herein.

Dr. Kaladevi Satish has no financial or proprietary interest in the materials presented herein.

Dr. David J. Spalton has no financial or proprietary interest in the materials presented herein.

Dr. Khiun F. Tjia is a consultant for Alcon and HOYA Surgical Optics.

Dr. Hiroshi Tsuneoka has no financial or proprietary interest in the materials presented herein.

Dr. Abhay R. Vasavada has no financial or proprietary interest in the materials presented herein.

Dr. Vaishali Vasavada has no financial or proprietary interest in the materials presented herein.

Dr. Viraj A. Vasavada has no financial or proprietary interest in the materials presented herein.

Dr. L. Felipe Vejarano has no financial or proprietary interest in the materials presented herein.

Dr. Robert Weinstock has no financial or proprietary interest in the materials presented herein.

INDEX

Abbott Medical Optics system. *See* WhiteStar Sovereign system
Accurus Surgical System, for gas infusion, 26
Acri.LISA toric multifocal lens, 176
Acri.Tec intraocular lenses, 167, 169-171, 178
AcrySof MA60AC lenses, 171
AcrySof ReStor lens, 173, 174
AcrySof SA60 series lenses, 165, 170-171
AcrySof Single-Piece lens insertion, 56-57
AcrySof SN60WF IQ lens, 110
air pumps, xxii, 24-29
    advantages of, 25
    vs. anesthesia type, 25-26
    continuous infusion with, 25
    for incomplete rhexis, 26-29
    in internal gas-forced infusion, 26
    method for, 25
    for microphakonit procedure, 128
    in Stellaris machine, 26, 62-64
    technique for, 24
Akahoshi Combo prechopper, 80
Akreos Adapt lens, 165
Akreos hydrophilic acrylic lenses, 178
Akreos M160 intraocular lens, 109, 167-169
Alcon Aspiration Bypass System, 6
Alcon INFINITI Vision System, 48, 50, 52
Alcon NeoSoniX system, 45-46
Alcon ReStor SN6AD3 lens, 173, 174
anesthesia
    surgery without, xxii, 25-26, 125, 152
    techniques for, xxiii
    for tilt and tumble technique, 115-116
    topical, air pump with, 25-26
    for WhiteStar system, 79
anterior capsule, in pediatric cataract, 145
anterior chamber
    torsional ultrasound effects on, 48
    vitrectomy of, for posterior capsule rupture, 185
anterior vented gas-forced infusion system, 26
antibiotics, before tilt and tumble technique, 115-116
antichamber collapser, 23, 128
aperture drape, for tilt and tumble technique, 116
aspheric intraocular lenses, 173, 174

aspiration
    instruments for, 42, 43
    in microphakonit procedure, 128, 129, 145
    for posterior capsule rupture, 184
    in sub-2-mm coaxial MICS, 109
    in tilt and tumble technique, 121-122
astigmatism
    induced, 17, 19, 20
    intraocular lenses for, 176, 177
    in tilt and tumble technique, 118-119
Attune Energy Management System, 66
Attune handpiece, 62, 66

balanced salt solution
    in hydrodissection, 40
    in tilt and tumble technique, 116
bent tips, 48-49
beveled tips, 49
biaxial MICS, xxiv-xxv
    for refractive cataract surgery, 177-179
bimanual MICS, xxiv-xxv, 9-10
    vs. coaxial MICS, 95, 106
    for floppy iris syndrome, 138
    fluidics in, 30-32
    in high myopia, 133
    history of, 105
    instruments for, 140
    intraocular cautery with, 140
    intraocular lenses for, 170-171
    after malignant melanoma excision, 138
    for mature cataract with zonular dialysis, 135
    with microcornea, 137
    with microphthalmos, 137
    needle sizes for, 90
    for posterior capsule rupture, 135
    for posterior polar cataract, 133-134
    for posterior subluxated cataract, 134
    in pseudoexfoliation, 135-136
    in punctured posterior capsule, 135
    after radial keratotomy, 139
    refractive lens exchange in, 138-139
    for rock-hard nuclei, 136-137
    switching hands in, 137
    three-port. *See* tilt and tumble technique
    torsional ultrasound with, 52
Bluetooth pedal, in Stellaris machine, 66-67
burst mode, for WhiteStar system, 71-72

INDEX

cannulas, for hydrodissection, 40
capsule
    anterior, in pediatric cataract, 145
    posterior. *See* posterior capsule
capsulorrhexis
    incomplete, air pump-assisted phaco for, 26-29
    instruments for, 38-39
    in microphakonit procedure, 130
    in sub-2-mm coaxial MICS, 107
    in tilt and tumble technique, 119
    transition from large to small, 89-90
carbachol, in tilt and tumble technique, 122
CASE (chamber automated stabilization environment), of WhiteStar, 75-77
cataract(s)
    dense
        bimanual MICS for, 135
        coaxial MICS for, 99-100
        tilt and tumble technique for, 114-115
        torsional ultrasound for, 52
    mature, bimanual MICS for, 135
    pediatric, 143-147
    posterior polar, 133-134
    posterior subluxated, 134
    soft, tilt and tumble technique for, 115
cautery, intraocular, 140
cavitation, 4-6, 65-66
chamber automated stabilization environment (CASE) model, of WhiteStar, 75-77
Chang cannula, 40
choppers
    Fat Boy, 109
    irrigating. *See* irrigating choppers
    for sub-2-mm coaxial MICS, 109
    Vejarano's, 38
chopstick forceps, 187
coaptation loss, 15, 16
coaxial MICS
    conventional, 95
    intraocular lenses for, 170-171
    1.8-mm, 10, 61-69
        advantages of, 61
        chamber stability in, 62-64
        fluidics in, 61-62
        foot pedal for, 66-67
        optimizing ultrasonic power for, 64-66
        power modulation in, 66
        StableChamber tubing for, 67-68
        technique for, 68
    2.2-mm, 95-103
        vs. bimanual MICS, 95
        vs. conventional coaxial phacoemulsification, 95
        for dense cataract, 99-100
        description of, 96
        first use of, 106
        incision for, 96
        instruments for, 96-97
        intraocular lens implantation in, 97
        for mitotic pupil, 100
        power modulation in, 97-98
        preoperative evaluation for, 100
        sphincter involving techniques for, 101
        sphincter sparing techniques for, 100
        technique for, 96-97
        torsional ultrasound with, 52, 54-55
    sub-2-mm, xxv, 105-111
        advantages of, 106
        aspiration in, 109
        vs. bimanual MICS, 106
        vs. historical incision size, 105-106
        instruments for, 106-109
        irrigation in, 109
        lenses for, 109-110
        phacodynamics for, 111
    unspecified size, fluidics in, 30
Collamer intraocular lens, 173, 174
compression cycle, 65
Concentrix pump, 6
continuous infusion, air pump with, 25
cornea
    aberrations profile of, 20
    incisions in. *See* incisions
    small, bimanual MICS with, 137
    topographic changes in, 17-19
cortical removal or aspiration
    in pediatric patients, 145
    for posterior capsule rupture, 184
    in tilt and tumble technique, 121-122
Crystalens lenses, 175, 176
cutter, vitreous, 9

Devine tip, for sub-2-mm coaxial MICS, 107
dialysis, of zonular apparatus, bimanual MICS for, 135
DigiFlow Pressurized Infusion, 26-29
draping, for tilt and tumble technique, 116
dual linear foot pedal, in Stellaris machine, 66-67
Dual Linear Millennium machine, for tilt and tumble technique, 121
Duckworth & Kent injector, 110
Duet system, for microphakonit procedure, 126, 128
duty cycle, for WhiteStar system, 71-72

Easy-Load inserter, of SofPort injector system, 161-162
Elastic Lens (STAAR), 159
Elastimide Lens (STAAR), 159
Ellips Transversal Phaco, 78-79

Emerald Series injector system, 159, 161
endothelium
    damage of, in tilt and tumble technique, 114
    defects of, tilt and tumble technique for, 115
    misalignment of, 13-14
energy, at phaco tip, 4-6
enhanced cavitation, 4, 5
epithelial misalignment, 13-14
evolution, of microincisional cataract surgery, xxi-xxvi
expansion cycle, 65
external gas-forced infusion, 128
extracapsular cataract extraction, 27-28, 185

Fat Boy chopper, 109
FAVIT technique, 190
floppy iris syndrome
    bimanual MICS for, 138, 178
    torsional ultrasound for, 55-56
flow pumps, 6
fluid inflow, modulating, 91
fluid outflow, modulating, 91-92
fluidics, 30-32
    for coaxial MICS, 61-62
    for microphakonit procedure, 126-128, 145
    in transition from large to small incisions, 90-92
foot pedal, in Stellaris machine, 66-67
forceps
    for capsulorrhexis, 38, 89-90
    chopstick, 187
    for pupillary membranes, 100
frequency, of machine, 3
frontal irrigation chopper, 41
Fusion Fluidics, with WhiteStar, 76, 78

glued intraocular lens, 189-190
glued sutureless vitrectomy, 150-152

handles, in Duet system, 128
hands, switching, in bimanual MICS, 137
healing, wound, 20, 21
heat, generation of, 65
high-infusion sleeve, 50
hooks, for pupil stretching, 101
horizontal chop, 8
horn, in phacoemulsification equipment, 46
Hoya Green Series injector systems, 162
Hoya iSert preloaded injector, 162
hybrid pumps, 6
hydration, stromal, 15
hydrodissection
    instruments for, 40
    in microphakonit procedure, 130
    in sub-2-mm coaxial MICS, 107
    in tilt and tumble technique, 119

ICE (increased control and efficiency) model, of WhiteStar, 73-74
incisions
    for coaxial MICS, 2.2-mm, 96
    instruments for, 37
    limbal relaxing, 118-119
    microinstruments for, 140
    for microphakonit procedure, 128-130, 145
    for pediatric cataract, 145
    for tilt and tumble technique, 117-119
    transition from large to small, 89-94
    for WhiteStar system, 79-80
inferior irrigation chopper, 41
INFINITI Vision System (Alcon), 48, 50, 52
infusion
    continuous, air pump with, 25
    internal gas-forced, 26
infusion sleeves
    for coaxial MICS, 96-97
    design of, 49-50
    for sub-2-mm coaxial MICS, 107, 109
    transition from large to small incisions, 90
injector systems, 157-163
    Hoya Green Series, 162
    Hoya preloaded, 162
    MicroSTAAR, 159
    Monarch III with D cartridge, 158
    preloaded, 158, 159, 162
    SofPort, 161-162
    STAAR, 158-159
    for sub-2-mm coaxial MICS, 110
    for ThinOptX rollable lens, 159, 160
    twisting and plunger method, 157-158
    Unfolder Emerald Series, 159, 161
    Unfolder Silver Series, 161
    uses of, 157
instrumentation, 37-43. *See also* specific instruments, eg, irrigating choppers; needle(s)
    for aspiration, 42, 43
    for bimanual MICS, 140
    for capsulorrhexis, 38-39
    for hydrodissection, 40
    for incision, 37
    irrigation choppers, 41
    knives, 38, 39
    needles, 40
    viscoelastics, 38
    for WhiteStar system, 80
Intelligent Phaco software, 109
internal gas-forced infusion, 26, 128
intraocular lens(es)
    aspheric, 173, 174
    evolution of, 105
    exchange of, 138-139
    foldable, 165-166
    glued, 189-190

insertion of
   in coaxial MICS, 97
   injectors for. *See* injector systems
   in microphakonit procedure, 145-146
   with posterior capsule rupture, 186-190
   in tilt and tumble technique, 122
   transition from large to small incisions, 92-93
microincisional, 165-172
   Acri.Tec, 167, 169-171
   Akreos M160, 167-169
   characteristics of, 169
   Lenstec ZR-1000, 169, 170
   performance of, 170-171
   for sub-2-mm coaxial MICS, 109-110
preloaded into injectors, 158, 159
refractive, 173-181
intraocular pressure, vs. wound architecture, 15, 17
IOLs. *See* intraocular lens(es)
iris hooks, for pupil stretching, 101
irrigating choppers, 23, 41, 80
   end-opening, 126
   for microphakonit procedure, 126-128
   side-opening, 126
irrigation
   in microphakonit procedure, 128, 129, 145
   in sub-2-mm coaxial MICS, 109
   in tilt and tumble technique, 113-114, 121-122

jackhammer effect, 4, 5, 46, 64-65

Kelman needle, for sub-2-mm coaxial MICS, 109
Kelman tip, for dense cataract, 100
keratotomy, radial, lens exchange after, 139
knives, 38, 39
   side-port, 106
   slit, 106-107
   for sub-2-mm coaxial MICS, 106-107

lancet, 38
lateral irrigation chopper, 41
leakage, postoperative, 20
lens, intraocular. *See* intraocular lens(es)
Lenstec ZR-1000 intraocular lens, 169, 170
light adjustable lenses, 178
limbal relaxing incision, in tilt and tumble technique, 118-119

machines, 3-11
   energy at phaco tip, 4-6
   for MICS, 9-10
   power generation for, 3

surge in, 6-9
vacuum sources for, 6
malignant melanoma, excision of, bimanual MICS after, 138
Malyugin ring
   for posterior capsule rupture, 187
   for pupil stretching, 101
mechanical impact, 65
melanoma, excision of, bimanual MICS after, 138
microcornea, bimanual MICS with, 137
MicroFlow tip, 40
microforceps, 80
microincisional cataract surgery, xxv
   advantages of, 176-178
   biaxial, xxiv-xxv
   bimanual. *See* bimanual MICS
   coaxial. *See* coaxial MICS
   in combination surgeries, 152-154
   0.7-mm. *See* microphakonit procedure (0.7-mm)
   for pediatric patients, 143-147
   refractive lenses for, 173-181
   sub-1-mm (0.7-mm), 125-132
   sub-2-mm, intraocular lenses for, 165-171
micrometer advance mechanism, in injectors, 157-158
microphakonit knife, 38
microphakonit procedure (0.7-mm), xxiv, 10, 125-132
   advantages of, 145-146
   air pump for, 128
   anterior capsule management in, 145
   anterior vitrectomy in, 146
   duet handles in, 128
   fluidics management in, 145
   glued 20-gauge sutureless vitrectomy with, 150-152
   history of, 125
   incisions in, 145
   indications for, 144-145
   intraocular lens insertion in, 145-146
   irrigating chopper for, 126-128
   irrigation aspiration system in, 128, 129
   vs. 0.9-mm technique, 128-131
   in no-anesthesia surgery, 152
   overview of, 126
   pars plana vitrectomy with, 149
   for pediatric patients, 143-147
   posterior capsule management in, 145-146
   preoperative evaluation for, 144
   trabeculectomy with, 152
   transconjunctival sutureless vitrectomy with, 150
microphthalmos, bimanual MICS with, 137
Microscissors, 38

MicroSTAAR injectors, 159
MicroTip, for very dense nuclei, 54
micro-Ultrata forceps, 38
MICS. *See* microincisional cataract surgery
Mini-Flared Kelman tip, 52
Mini-Flared MicroTip, 48
miotic pupil, coaxial MICS for, 100-101
Monarch III with D cartridge, 158
myopia, high, bimanual MICS in, 133

Nano Sleeve (Alcon), 52, 96, 107, 109
Nanopoint injector system, 158
nanotip needle, 40
needle(s), 40
    energy at tip, 4-6
    for microphakonit procedure, 126
    sizes of, 92
    for sub-2-mm coaxial MICS, 109
    transition from large to small, 90, 92
NeoSoniX system (Alcon), 45-46
Nichamin Age Adjusted and Pachymetry Adjusted nomogram, 118-119
nucleus
    dense, torsional ultrasound for, 53-54
    drop of, 190
    removal of, in pediatric patients, 145
    rock-hard, bimanual MICS for, 136-137

Oertli Smart tip, for sub-2-mm coaxial MICS, 107, 109
ophthalmic viscosurgical devices, 80
optical coherence tomography, for wound evaluation, 13
Optical Quality Analysis System, 20
ORange lens (WaveTec), 179
OZil torsional handpiece and software, 45-46, 50, 53

Packard needle, for sub-2-mm coaxial MICS, 109
pars plana vitrectomy, MICS with, 149
pedal, foot, in Stellaris machine, 66-67
pediatric cataracts, 143-147
    clinical features of, 143
    MICS for
        advantages of, 145-146
        indications for, 144-145
        preoperative evaluation for, 144
        technique for, 145-146
        technology for, 143
    syndromes associated with, 144
perfluorocarbon, for dropped nucleus, 190
peristaltic pumps, in WhiteStar system, 78
phaco chop, 7
photography, shadow field, 64
plungers, in injector systems, 157-158

posterior capsule
    management of, in microphakonit procedure, 145-146
    punctured, bimanual MICS for, 135
    rupture of, 183-192
        anterior bimanual vitrectomy for, 185
        anterior chamber clearance for, 185
        bimanual MICS for, 135
        conversion to extracapsular extraction for, 185
        dry cortical aspiration for, 184
        intraocular lens insertion with, 186-190
        nucleus drop in, 190
        reducing parameters for, 184
        sequelae of, 191
        signs of, 183
        torsional ultrasound for, 56
        viscoexpression for, 185
        wound suturing for, 185
posterior polar cataract, bimanual MICS for, 133-134
posterior subluxated cataract, bimanual MICS for, 134
Pouiseuille's equation, 91
power
    generation of, 3
    modulation of, 66, 97-98
    optimizing, 64-66
prechopping device, 53, 80
preloaded injectors, 158, 159
presbyopia, intraocular lenses for, 173-176
proportional-integral-differential computer algorithms, 64
pseudoexfoliation, bimanual MICS in, 135-136
pulse mode, for WhiteStar system, 71
Pulser Power, 66
pumps. *See also* air pumps
    peristaltic, 78
    vacuum, 6
    Venturi, 78, 121
    in WhiteStar system, 78
punctured posterior capsule, bimanual MICS for, 135
pupil
    large, tilt and tumble technique for, 115
    small
        coaxial MICS for, 100-101
        tilt and tumble technique for, 115
    stretching of, 101

radial keratotomy, lens exchange after, 139
refractive cataract surgery, MICS with, 173-181
    lenses for, 173-179
    technique for, 177-178
ReStor SN6AD3 lens, 173, 174

ReZoom intraocular lens, 175, 178
rhexis. *See* capsulorrhexis
rock-hard nuclei, bimanual MICS for, 136-137

scissors, 38, 101
shadow field photography, 64
side-port instruments, for sub-2-mm coaxial MICS, 109
side-port knife, 106
Signature system, of WhiteStar, 76, 78
Silver Series injector system, 161
Sinskey tip, 80
sleeveless microphacoemulsification, three-port. *See* tilt and tumble technique
sleeves, infusion. *See* infusion sleeves
slit knife, 106-107
Smart IOL, 167, 169
sodium hyaluronate, 80
SofPort injector systems, 161-162
Sovereign peristaltic pump, 6
sphincter
    coaxial MICS techniques involving, 101
    sparing of, in coaxial MICS, 100
sphincterotomy, for small pupil, 101
STAAR Collamer intraocular lens, 173, 174
STAAR injector systems, 158-159
STAAR Toric intraocular lens, 176, 177
StableChamber tubing and fluidics module, 63-64, 67-68
Stellaris DigiFlow Pressurized Infusion, 26
Stellaris machine, for coaxial MICS, 61-69
    advantages of, 61
    chamber stability in, 62-64
    fluidics in, 61-62
    foot pedal for, 66-67
    optimizing ultrasonic power for, 64-66
    power modulation in, 66
    StableChamber tubing for, 67-68
    technique for, 68
straight tips, 48-49
stroke length, of machine, 3
stromal hydration, 15
sulcus, intraocular lens insertion into, 186-187
suprascapular phacoemulsification. *See* tilt and tumble technique
surge
    causes of, 62
    control of, 6-9, 32, 62
    transition from large to small incisions, 92
sustained cavitation, 4-6
sutureless vitrectomy, MICS with, 150-152
switching hands, in bimanual MICS, 137
synechiae, 100
syringe advance mechanism, in injectors, 157-158

tear, posterior capsule. *See* posterior capsule, rupture of
TECNIS lenses, 173-176, 178
terminology, for MICS, xv
tetracaine drops, before tilt and tumble technique, 115-116
ThinOptX rollable lens, injector systems for, 159, 160
ThinOptX Ultrachoice lens, 167, 170, 171
three-port bimanual sleeveless microphacoemulsification. *See* tilt and tumble technique
tilt and tumble technique, 113-124
    advantages of, 114
    capsulorrhexis in, 119
    cortical removal in, 121-122
    hydrodissection in, 119
    incisions in, 117-119
    indications for, 114-115
    intraocular lens insertion in, 122
    overview of, 113-114
    phacoemulsification in, 120-121
    preoperative preparation for, 115-116
    procedure for, 117-122
    skills for, 117
tips
    bent, 48-49
    beveled, 49
    energy at, 4-6
    nanotip, 40
    straight, 48-49
    for sub-2-mm coaxial MICS, 107, 109
    for torsional ultrasound, 48-51, 53-54
    types of, 49-50
topical anesthesia, air pump with, 25-26
torsional ultrasound, 45-59
    for AcrySof Single-Piece lens insertion, 56-57
    advantages of, 52
    anterior chamber stability with, 48
    for coaxial MICS, 54-55, 98
    for complex cases, 54-56
    vs. conventional ultrasound, 46-47
    for dense cataracts, 52
    for dense nuclei, 53-54
    for floppy iris syndrome, 55-56
    history of, 45
    innovative prechopping device for, 53
    for posterior capsule tear, 56
    software for, 50
    tip design and, 48-51, 53-54
    for zonular weakness, 55
trabeculectomy, MICS with, 152
transcleral pars plana vitrectomy, MICS with, 149

transconjunctival sutureless vitrectomy, MICS with, 150
transient cavitation, 4
transition, to MICS, 89-94
    fluidics, 90-92
    instrumentation, 89-90
    intraocular lens insertion, 92-93
    needles, 9, 90
transverse ultrasound, 78-79, 98
triamcinolone acetonide, for vitrectomy visualization, 185
tubing, in Stellaris machine, 63-64, 67-68
twisting and plunging method, for lens insertion, 157-158

Ultra Sleeve, 96, 107, 109
Ultrachoice lens, 167, 170, 171
Ultrachopper, 53
ultrasound, torsional. *See* torsional ultrasound
Unfolder Emerald Series injector system, 159, 161
Unfolder Silver Series injector system, 161
Utrata forceps, 100

vacuum pumps, 6
Variable WhiteStar, 73, 81-84
Vejarano's choppers, 38
Venturi pumps, 78, 121
vertical chop, 9
viscoelastics, 38
    for sub-2-mm coaxial MICS, 107
    for synechiae, 100
    for tilt and tumble technique, 119, 120
viscoexpression, for posterior capsule rupture, 185
viscomydriasis, 100
vitrectomy, 9
    anterior
        in microphakonit procedure, for pediatric patients, 146
        for posterior capsule rupture, 185

    glued sutureless, MICS with, 150-152
    pars plana, MICS with, 149
    transconjunctival sutureless, MICS with, 150
WaveTec ORange lens, 179
WhiteStar Sovereign system (Abbott Medical Optics), 71-85
    anesthesia for, 79
    CASE (chamber automated stabilization environment), 75-77
    dual-pump technology for, 78
    Ellips Transversal, 78-79
    ICE model, 73-74
    incisions for, 79-80
    instruments for, 80
    micropulse technology of, 71-73
    ophthalmic viscosurgical devices for, 80-84
    Signature, 76, 78
    software settings for, 80-84
    technique for, 79-84
    Variable model, 73, 81-84
wireless foot pedal, in Stellaris machine, 66-67
wound
    architecture of, vs. intraocular pressure, 15, 17
    evaluation of, 13
    extension of, 15
    healing of, 20, 21
    without extension of, 13-15

Xcelens Idea lenses, 165

zonular dialysis, in mature cataract, bimanual MICS for, 135
zonular weakness, torsional ultrasound for, 55

Wait...There's More!

SLACK Incorporated's Health Care Books and Journals offers a wide selection of books in the field of Ophthalmology. We are dedicated to providing important works that educate, inform and improve the knowledge of our customers. Don't miss out on our other informative titles that will enhance your collection.

Fundus Fluorescein and Indocyanine Green Angiography: A Textbook and Atlas
Amar Agarwal MS, FRCS, FRCOphth

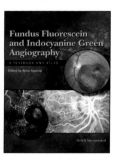

288 pp, Hard Cover, 2008, ISBN 13 978-1-55642-787-9, Order# 67875, **$139.95**

Fundus Fluorescein and Indocyanine Green Angiography is a complete and detailed reference that comprehensively covers fluorescein angiography, the more recent and advancing indocyanine green angiography and their effectiveness in identifying and evaluating various retinal diseases.

Refractive Surgery Nightmares:
Conquering Refractive Surgery Catastrophes
Amar Agarwal MS, FRCS, FRCOphth

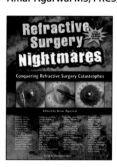

424 pp, Hard Cover, 2007, ISBN 13 978-1-55642-788-6, Order# 67883, **$184.95**

Dr. Amar Agarwal, along with contributions from 67 of today's leading refractive surgery experts, explains all there is to know about refractive surgery techniques in *Refractive Surgery Nightmares* to help you stay in control when facing unique surgical challenges.

Dry Eye: A Practical Guide to Ocular Surface Disorders and Stem Cell Surgery
Amar Agarwal MS, FRCS, FRCOphth

392 pp, Hard Cover, 2006, ISBN 13 978-1-55642-751-0, Order# 67514, **$109.95**

Dry eye and ocular surface disorders are complex conditions with multiple modes of treatment. Navigate your way through the perplexities with *Dry Eye*.

Handbook of Ophthalmology
Amar Agarwal MS, FRCS, FRCOphth

752 pp, Soft Cover, 2006, ISBN 13 978-1-55642-685-8, Order# 66852, **$69.95**

The *Handbook of Ophthalmology*, edited by Dr. Amar Agarwal, is a pocket-sized, ready reference book that provides a compact review of diagnostic eye disorders.

Phaco Nightmares:
Conquering Cataract Catastrophes
Amar Agarwal MS, FRCS, FRCOphth

464 pp, Hard Cover, 2006, ISBN 13 978-1-55642-772-5, Order# 67727, **$184.95**

Even the most experienced cataract surgeon can encounter stressful situations in the operating room. Be prepared to manage unavoidable complications with *Phaco Nightmares*.

Video Atlas of Advanced Ophthalmic Surgeries
Amar Agarwal MS, FRCS, FRCOphth

DVD, 2010, ISBN 13 978-1-55642-878-4, Order# 68784, **$99.95**

With 116 videos, this video based textbook contains nearly 10 hours of state of the art video teaching.

Video Atlas of Basic Ophthalmic Surgeries
Amar Agarwal MS, FRCS, FRCOphth

DVD, 2010, ISBN 13 978-1-55642-877-7, Order# 68777, **$99.95**

With 129 videos, this video based textbook contains nearly 10 hours of state of the art video teaching.

Please visit **www.slackbooks.com** to order any of the above titles!
24 Hours a Day...7 Days a Week!

Attention Industry Partners!

Whether you are interested in buying multiple copies of a book, chapter reprints, or looking for something new and different — we are able to accommodate your needs.

MULTIPLE COPIES

At attractive discounts starting for purchases as low as 25 copies for a single title, SLACK Incorporated will be able to meet all of your needs.

CHAPTER REPRINTS

SLACK Incorporated is able to offer the chapters you want in a format that will lead to success. Bound with an attractive cover, use the chapters that are a fit specifically for your company. Available for quantities of 100 or more.

CUSTOMIZE

SLACK Incorporated is able to create a specialized custom version of any of our products specifically for your company.

Please contact the Marketing Communications Director for further details on multiple copy purchases, chapter reprints or custom printing at 1-800-257-8290 or 1-856-848-1000.

*Please note all conditions are subject to change.

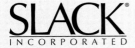

Health Care Books and Journals • 6900 Grove Road • Thorofare, NJ 08086

1-800-257-8290
Fax: 1-856-848-6091
E-mail: orders@slackinc.com

www.slackbooks.com